DOSAGES and SOLUTIONS
edition 4

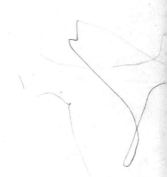

DOSAGES and SOLUTIONS
edition 4

DOROTHY M. BLUME, R.N., M.S.N.

ASSOCIATE PROFESSOR
THE UNIVERSITY OF TEXAS AT AUSTIN
SCHOOL OF NURSING
AUSTIN, TEXAS

EMILY F. CORNETT, R.N., PH.D.

ASSOCIATE PROFESSOR
THE UNIVERSITY OF TEXAS AT AUSTIN
SCHOOL OF NURSING
AUSTIN, TEXAS

F. A. DAVIS COMPANY Philadelphia

Library of Congress Cataloging in Publication Data

Blume, Dorothy M.
    Dosages and solutions.

    Includes index.
    1. Drugs—Dosage—Problems, exercises, etc.
2. Solutions (Pharmacy)—Problems, exercises, etc.
I. Cornett, Emily F., 1932–   . II. Title. [DNLM:
1. Drugs—Administration and dosage.   2. Solutions—
Laboratory manuals.   QV 25 B658d]
RM145.B55   1983   615′.14   83-7413
ISBN 0-8036-0953-1

PREFACE

Dosages and Solutions is written primarily for nursing students. However, it will also be of value for in-service education programs, for refresher courses for inactive nurses, and as a desk reference for nurses who administer medications wherever they are employed. An early introduction to classroom laboratory problems using actual drugs and equipment is suggested for students using one book.

The book offers a practical approach to the preparation of drug dosages and solutions. Suggested methods of doing calculations have been reduced to a few variations of direct ratio and proportion. However, examples were selected to reflect the realistic and often difficult problems encountered in preparing drugs and solutions for administration.

This edition features revisions and additions of new material throughout the text. Changes include clarification of weight to volume equivalents, problems rarely encountered, and calculations when determined by the nurse's judgment. All outdated drugs and problems have been deleted. Young's, Fried's, and Clark's rules are stated but not used for examples or practice problems. Recalculation of reconstitution problems to provide the ordered dose in one milliliter has also been deleted.

The administration of insulin section, illustrations of syringes, and calculation of children's dosages have been updated. The section of intravenous medications has been revised to reflect current equipment and procedures.

Additions include alternate ways of stating ratios and proportions; use of oral syringes and calibrated medicine droppers; actual drug labels; calculation of fluid loss or gain; more example, practice, and review problems; the use of ointments and suppositories; more detailed explanation of the concept of drug displacements; additional reasonable answers and how solutions were derived; use of the nomogram; conversion from pounds to kilograms; discussion and illustrations of currently used intravenous administration sets and equipment; summary of steps in the administration of fluids and drugs intravenously; the calculation of calories in intravenous fluids; and the calculation of fluid maintenance needs. Centigrade to Fahrenheit equivalents and tables of Roman and Arabic numerals have been added to the arithmetic pretest, explanation section, practice problems, and an entirely new arithmetic post-test.

We wish to express our sincere appreciation to students and to faculty members in schools of nursing who have used this workbook, whose comments and helpful suggestions have guided this revision. We especially want to thank those nurses and pharmacists in local hospitals and in teaching institutions for their contributions to this edition.

Dorothy M. Blume
Emily F. Cornett

CONTENTS

CHAPTER 1

INTRODUCTION

In many hospitals the pharmacy provides nursing units with medications in what is called "unit dose." This means that drugs are available to the nurse in the amount ordered to be given. Therefore, little or no calculation of dosages is necessary.

However, on some units in most hospitals, such as the Emergency Room, Intensive Care and Coronary Care Units, nurses must calculate and prepare many medications. In most small hospitals they must do so on all units.

Working dosage problems involves the calculation of the correct dosage to be administered to the patient, usually either orally or parenterally, in order to give the prescribed amount of a drug. Usually the physician orders the drug in numbers of grains, grams, or other units of *weight* measure. To administer the correct dosage, nurses often need to convert this order to a number of tablets, capsules, minims, drams, ounces, milliliters, or other units of *volume or capacity* measure. A single ratio and proportion formula (hereafter referred to as Formula B, see p. 5) can be used to work all dosage problems.

Doing solutions problems involves determining how to prepare solutions, for either oral or topical use. There are two variations of solutions problems, but both can be solved by using Formula B.

In solving either dosage or solutions problems a second ratio and proportion formula (hereafter referred to as Formula A, see p. 5) may be used to determine equivalent values whenever necessary. This additional initial step may be necessary in order to limit the different units of measure in any proportion to two units of measure. One can say, for example, that 4 wheels:1 car = 8 wheels:2 cars. One cannot say, however, that 4 wheels:1 car = 8 wheels:2 bicycles. Therefore, if the physician orders aspirin grains 10 and the available tablets are labeled "0.3 gram," Formula A would be used first to convert either grains 10 to its gram equivalent or to convert 0.3 gram to its grains equivalent. Then, when using Formula B to determine how many tablets to give, tablets would be one unit of measure and either grains or grams the other unit of measure. A grain is an apothecaries' system unit of measure; a gram is a metric system unit of measure.

An arithmetic review is given in Appendix C. This review may be used as a pretest if desired by the user or instructor. Answers to these and all practice problems are found at the end of this book and will provide immediate knowledge of results to the users, which should enhance learning.

SYSTEMS OF MEASUREMENT

The American colonists brought to this country the use of the apothecaries' system of weights and measures which was then being used in England. England is now adopting use of the metric system which has long been the single lawful system in most European countries. Since World War II there has been a growing tendency in the United States for doctors to order and for pharmaceutical companies to label drugs with the metric system units of measure. Learning to administer drugs would be greatly simplified if only the metric system were used. Until that time, however, nurses need to know about three systems of measurement: the apothecaries', the metric, and the household systems. More complete tables and explanations of these three systems and approximate equivalents among the systems may be found in Appendix A. Further explanations are included throughout the workbook.

One thing should be emphasized before anyone becomes discouraged from consulting these lengthy tables. Almost all the equivalents that nurses ever need to know can be determined by using ratio and proportion with the few equivalents listed in Table 1. Learn ratio and proportion and these equivalents backwards, forwards, and crosswise; then mastering dosage and solutions will be simple.

It is customary to use regular fractions for the apothecaries' system and decimal fractions for the metric system. *To minimize the danger of error, a zero is placed before the decimal point when writing a fraction of a metric unit.*

Sometimes symbols are used to express apothecaries' units of measure. The most commonly used apothecaries' symbols are ʒ for dram and ℥ for ounce. Also, when using the apothecaries' units the numerical value or the quantity of a unit is often expressed in Roman numerals, usually in lower case letters. For example, five grains may be written as grains v; four drams as ʒ iv and six ounces as ℥ vi. For review see Appendix A.

Occasionally household measures are used for ordering dosages of medications. The quantity may be written in either Arabic or Roman numerals. For example, 15 drops may be written as 15 gtts. or as gtts. xv. Gtts. is an acceptable abbreviation for drops. See Appendix B for a list of abbreviations commonly used in the administration of medications.

TABLE 1. Most frequently used approximate equivalents

WEIGHT UNITS			FLUID UNITS		
HOUSE-HOLD	METRIC	APOTHE-CARIES'	APOTHE-CARIES'	METRIC	HOUSE-HOLD
	1 gram or 1000 milli-grams or 1,000,000 micro-grams	15 or 16 grains	15 or 16 minims	1 milliliter	15 or 16 drops
2 table-spoons or 3 dessert spoons or 6 tea-spoons	30 or 32 grams	1 ounce or 8 drams	1 fluid ounce or 8 fluid drams	30 or 32 milliliters	2 table-spoons or 3 dessert spoons or 6 tea-spoons
			1 pint or 16 fluid ounces	500 milli-liters	2 glasses
	1 kilogram or 1000 grams	2.2 or 2.3 pounds (imperial or avoir-dupois— not apothe-caries')	1 quart	1000 milli-liters or 1 liter	4 glasses
			1 gallon	4000 milli-liters	

RATIO AND PROPORTION

A ratio is the same as a fraction and can be expressed in algebraic form (1:2) or as a regular fraction (1/2). Either way, the relationship is stated as "one is to two."

A proportion is an equation of equal fractions or ratios. For example, the ratios 1/2 and 4/8 are equal, or "one is to two as four is to eight" (1:2::4:8) or "one is to two equals four is to eight" (1:2 = 4:8).

The first and fourth terms of a proportion are called the extremes and the second and third terms the means. In solving these equations the product of the means equals the product of the extremes.

$$\text{Means}$$

$$\text{First Term}:\text{Second Term} = \text{Third Term}:\text{Fourth Term}$$

$$\text{Extremes}$$

or

$$\text{means}$$

$$1:2 = 4:8 \qquad \begin{array}{l} 1 \times 8 = 8 \\ 2 \times 4 = 8 \end{array}$$

$$\text{extremes}$$

The terms of the two ratios of a proportion must correspond in relative value. For example, small is to small as large is to large, or small is to large as small is to large.

$$1:2 = 4:8 \qquad \text{small}:\text{small} = \text{large}:\text{large}?$$
$$\textit{or}$$
$$\text{small}:\text{large} = \text{small}:\text{large}?$$

This correspondence, which is confusing enough when only numerical values are used, is more confusing when numerical values plus two units of measure are involved, as in dosage and solutions problems. For example, if 15 grains equals 1 gram, 30 grains equals how many grams?

$$15 \text{ gr.}:1 \text{ Gm.} = 30 \text{ gr.}:x \text{ Gm.}$$
$$15\,x = 30$$
$$x = 2 \text{ Gm.}; \text{ therefore, 30 gr. equals 2 Gm.}$$

or

$$15 \text{ gr.}:1 \text{ Gm.} = 30 \text{ gr.}:2 \text{ Gm.}$$

Disregarding numerical values, the ratios in the above proportion correspond—small:large = small:large—because grains are smaller units of measure than grams. However, numerical values cannot be disregarded. Both the relative value of the units of measure and the relative value of the quantities of these units of measure must be considered. Otherwise, even when using the correct numerical values, the product of the means *may not equal* the product of the extremes, as shown below.

$$2 \times 30 = 60$$

$$15 \text{ gr.}:2 \text{ Gm.} = 30 \text{ gr.}:1 \text{ Gm.}$$

$$15 \times 1 = 15$$

Unless the proportion is stated properly the solution to the problem will be *incorrect*, as shown below.

$$15 \text{ gr.}:x \text{ Gm.} = 30 \text{ gr.}:1 \text{ Gm.}$$
$$30 x = 15$$
$$x = 0.5 \text{ Gm.; therefore, } 30 \text{ gr. equals } 0.5 \text{ Gm.}$$

There are several possible ways, as shown below, to state *correctly* any one proportion.

$$15 \text{ gr.}:1 \text{ Gm.} = 30 \text{ gr.}:2 \text{ Gm.}$$
or
$$15 \text{ gr.}:30 \text{ gr.} = 1 \text{ Gm.}:2 \text{ Gm.}$$
or
$$30 \text{ gr.}:2 \text{ Gm.} = 15 \text{ gr.}:1 \text{ Gm.}$$
or
$$30 \text{ gr.}:15 \text{ gr.} = 2 \text{ Gm.}:1 \text{ Gm.}$$
or
$$1 \text{ Gm.}:2 \text{ Gm.} = 15 \text{ gr.}:30 \text{ gr.}$$
or
$$1 \text{ Gm.}:15 \text{ gr.} = 2 \text{ Gm.}:30 \text{ gr.}$$
or
$$2 \text{ Gm.}:1 \text{ Gm.} = 1 \text{ Gm.}:15 \text{ gr.}$$
or
$$2 \text{ Gm.}:30 \text{ gr.} = 1 \text{ Gm.}:15 \text{ gr.}$$

There are just as many possible ways to state *incorrectly* any one proportion.

KNOWN VALUES FORMULAS

Avoid confusion by starting every proportion with a ratio of two *known values*, for example, 15 grains:1 gram (*known* equivalents) or 5 grains:1 tablet (dosage in a certain unit of measure which is *known* to be available for administration). Next, when using Formulas A and B make certain that the unit of measure of the third term is the same as that in the first term and that the unit of measure of the fourth term is the same as that in the second term.

Formula A   *known equivalents*
(conversions) $15 \text{ gr.}:1 \text{ Gm.} = x \text{ gr.}:0.5 \text{ Gm.}$

Formula B   *known amounts*
(dosages) $5 \text{ gr.}:1 \text{ tablet} = 15 \text{ gr.}:x \text{ tablet(s)}$

As stated above, in all dosage and solutions problems there may be two, but no more than two, different units of measure in addition to numerical values. Label every term in the proportion with a unit of measure. Forget these units of measure when multiplying means and extremes. Finally, label x, the unknown quantity, with the appropriate unit of measure.

Examples:

PROBLEM 1. Determine the gr. equivalent of 0.5 Gm.

SOLUTION: FORMULA A

known equivalents   unknown equivalents
$$15 \text{ gr.:1 Gm.} = x \text{ gr.:0.5 Gm.}$$
$$1 x = 7 \; 1/2$$
$$x = 7 \; 1/2 \text{ gr.}$$

PROBLEM 2. Determine how many tablets to administer when the order is for aspirin gr. xv and the available tablets are gr. v each.

SOLUTION: FORMULA B

known amounts   unknown amount
(available for use)   (ordered)   (needed)
dosage:amount = dosage:amount
$$5 \text{ gr.:1 tablet} = 15 \text{ gr.:}x \text{ tablet(s)}$$
$$5 x = 15$$
$$x = 3 \text{ tablets}$$

Note that the first ratio or the first and the second terms in the proportion above are all *known* values. All dosage and solutions problems can be solved by using variations of Formula B. By using the few equivalents listed in Table 1 and Formula A, one can determine almost all other equivalents nurses ever need to know.

DETERMINING EQUIVALENT VALUES

Three examples of determining equivalent values by using Formula A are presented below, along with discussions of commonly encountered problems. Additional help in determining equivalents is presented later with the answers to the various types of dosage and solutions problems.

Examples

PROBLEM 1. 1 gr. = ? mg.

SOLUTION 1

known equivalents   unknown equivalents
$$15 \text{ gr.:1000 mg.} = 1 \text{ gr.:}x \text{ mg.}$$
$$15 x = 1000$$
$$x = 66.67 \text{ mg.}$$

or

SOLUTION 2

$$16 \text{ gr.}:1000 \text{ mg.} = 1 \text{ gr.}:x \text{ mg.}$$
$$16 x = 1000$$
$$x = 62.5 \text{ mg.}$$

If one remembers the numbers 60, 64, and 65 mg. given in equivalent tables and remembers that 15 or 16 gr. = 1 Gm. = 1000 mg., one can readily see that 1 gr. = 60, 64, or 65 mg. and that 1 mg. = 1/60, 1/64, or 1/65 gr.

$$1 \text{ Gm.} = 1000 \text{ mg.} = 15 \text{ or } 16 \text{ gr.}$$
$$60, 64, \text{ or } 65 \text{ mg.} = 1 \text{ gr.}$$
$$1 \text{ mg.} = 1/60, 1/64, \text{ or } 1/65 \text{ gr.}$$

Any of these values is accurate enough for calculation of dosages. Often the choice of one over the other two enables division of numerators and denominators by the same number in order to reduce these parts of fractions to smaller numerical values which are more likely to be the same values as the ordered dosages.

PROBLEM 2.   32 mg. = ? gr.

SOLUTION 1

$$1 \text{ gr.}:64 \text{ mg.} = x \text{ gr.}:32 \text{ mg.}$$
$$64 x = 32$$
$$x = 1/2 \text{ gr.}$$

rather than

SOLUTION 2

$$1 \text{ gr.}:60 \text{ mg.} = x \text{ gr.}:32 \text{ mg.}$$
$$60 x = 32$$
$$x = 32/60 = 8/15 \text{ gr.}$$

If the physician's order is for 32 mg. of a certain drug and the tablets are labeled in gr., use 1 gr.:64 mg. = x gr.:32 mg. If the physician's order is for 30 mg. of this drug, use 1 gr.:60 mg. = x gr.:30 mg., because whether the doctor orders 30 mg. or 32 mg. the available tablets are probably labeled "gr. 1," "gr. 1/2," or "gr. 1/4." Of course, the tablets may be labeled "30 mg.," or "32 mg.," or possibly "0.03 Gm.," or "0.032 Gm."

PROBLEM 3.   Nembutal 100 mg. = Nembutal ? gr.

SOLUTION 1

$$15 \text{ gr.}:1000 \text{ mg.} = x \text{ gr.}:100 \text{ mg.}$$
$$1000 x = 1500$$
$$x = 1 \text{ } 1/2 \text{ gr.}$$

SOLUTION 2

$$1 \text{ gr.}:65 \text{ mg.} = x \text{ gr.}:100 \text{ mg.}$$
$$65 x = 100$$
$$x = 1 \text{ } 35/65 \text{ gr.}$$

7

SOLUTION 3

$$1 \text{ gr.}:60 \text{ mg.} = x \text{ gr.}:100 \text{ mg.}$$
$$60x = 100$$
$$x = 1 \ 2/3 \text{ gr.}$$

SOLUTION 4

$$1 \text{ gr.}:64 \text{ mg.} = x \text{ gr.}:100 \text{ mg.}$$
$$64x = 100$$
$$x = 1 \ 9/16 \text{ gr.}$$

There are a few basic rules that apply to all problems. *One is that no more than a 10% margin of difference between ordered and administered dosages may be considered safe.* For example, if the physician orders Nembutal 100 mg., no more than 110 mg. or no less than 90 mg. should be administered. This margin of difference allows for variances in determined dosages which may result from the particular equivalent values used. For example, Nembutal may be available in capsules gr. 3/4 and gr. 1 1/2. If gr. 1 = 60 mg., then gr. 1 1/2 = 90 mg., and 1 tablet labeled "gr. 1 1/2" may safely be given. This and most problems can be solved many different ways, giving slightly different but accurate answers.

PROBLEM 4.   1 teaspoon = ? milliliters

SOLUTION 1

$$6 \text{ tsp.}:(1 \text{ oz.}) \ 30 \text{ ml.} = 1 \text{ tsp.}:x \text{ ml.}$$
$$6x = 30$$
$$x = 5 \text{ ml.}$$

SOLUTION 2

$$6 \text{ tsp.}:(1 \text{ oz.}) \ 32 \text{ ml.} = 1 \text{ tsp.}:x \text{ ml.}$$
$$6x = 32$$
$$x = 5 \ 1/3 \text{ ml.}$$

PROBLEM 5.   1 dram = ? milliliters

SOLUTION 1

$$8 \text{ dr.}:(1 \text{ oz.}) \ 32 \text{ ml.} = 1 \text{ dr.}:x \text{ ml.}$$
$$8x = 32$$
$$x = 4 \text{ ml.}$$

SOLUTION 2

$$8 \text{ dr.}:(1 \text{ oz.}) \ 30 \text{ ml.} = 1 \text{ dr.}:x \text{ ml.}$$
$$8x = 30$$
$$x = 3 \ 3/4 \text{ ml.}$$

It is suggested that the equivalents 1 teaspoon equals 5 milliliters and 1 dram equals 4 milliliters be used when calculating dosages.

PROBLEM 6.   1 tablespoon = ? milliliters

SOLUTION 1

$$2 \text{ Tbsp.}:(1 \text{ oz.}) \ 30 \text{ ml.} = 1 \text{ Tbsp.}:x \text{ ml.}$$
$$2x = 30$$
$$x = 15 \text{ ml.}$$

SOLUTION 2

$$2 \text{ Tbsp.:}(1 \text{ oz.}) \; 32 \text{ ml.} = 1 \text{ Tbsp.:} x \text{ ml.}$$
$$2x = 32$$
$$x = 16 \text{ ml.}$$

PROBLEM 7.   1 tablespoon = ? drams

SOLUTION

$$(1 \text{ oz.}) \; 32 \text{ ml.:} 8 \text{ dr.} = 16 \text{ ml.:} x \text{ dr.}$$
$$32x = 128$$
$$x = 4 \text{ dr.}$$

If the number of milliliters in a tablespoon is not known, first determine this as in problem 6 above.

PROBLEM 8.   20 pounds = ? kilograms

SOLUTION

$$2.2 \text{ lbs.:} 1 \text{ kg.} = 20 \text{ lbs.:} x \text{ kg.}$$
$$2.2x = 20$$
$$x = 9.09 \text{ or } 9.1 \text{ kg.}$$

ALTERNATIVE WAYS OF STATING RATIOS AND PROPORTIONS

Other methods of setting up the ratios may be used by those who are more familiar with one of these methods. One of the most commonly used alternative methods is to state the first and third terms of the previous method as numerators and the second and fourth terms as denominators. In other words, the ratios are expressed as regular fractions. For example, 15 gr.:1000 mg. = x gr.:100 mg. can be shown as follows:

known equivalents $\left[\dfrac{15 \text{ gr.}}{1000 \text{ mg.}} = \dfrac{x \text{ gr.}}{100 \text{ mg.}} \right]$ unknown equivalents

$$1000x = 1500$$
$$x = 1.5 \text{ or } 1 \; 1/2 \text{ gr.}$$

Or, five grains is to one tablet as 15 grains is to how many tablets?

known amounts $\left[\dfrac{5 \text{ gr.}}{1 \text{ tablet}} = \dfrac{15 \text{ gr.}}{x \text{ tablets}} \right]$ unknown amount

$$5x = 15$$
$$x = 3 \text{ tablets}$$

To solve these fractional equations cross multiply diagonally. Whichever way the ratios are stated, the product of the means equals the product of the extremes.

means

15 gr.:1000 mg. = x gr.:100 mg.

extremes

9

or

$$\begin{array}{c} \text{extreme} \\ \text{mean} \end{array} \quad \frac{15 \text{ gr.}}{1000 \text{ mg.}} = \frac{x \text{ gr.}}{100 \text{ mg.}} \quad \begin{array}{c} \text{mean} \\ \text{extreme} \end{array}$$

Some may prefer to use one of the several variations of the formula of desired dose over the available dose times the unit of measurement of the available dose equals the amount to give. The unit of measurement of the available dose is the numerator over an implied denominator of one. This method will not be used in this book because the authors have found that students make more errors with this method and it cannot be used for all types of problem calculations. It is included as a review for those who have already learned this way of solving problems.

$$\frac{\text{Ordered dose}}{\text{Available dose}} \times \begin{array}{c} \text{Unit of measurement} \\ \text{of available dose} \end{array} = \begin{array}{c} \text{Amount to give in} \\ \text{same unit of} \\ \text{measurement} \end{array}$$

or

$$\frac{15 \text{ gr.}}{5 \text{ gr.}} \times 1 \text{ tablet} = \text{Amount to give}$$

$$\frac{15 \text{ gr.}}{5 \text{ gr.}} \times \frac{1 \text{ tablet}}{1} = \text{Amount to give}$$

$$\frac{15}{5} = 3 \text{ tablets}$$

$$\frac{\text{D (desired dose)}}{\text{H (on hand dose)}} \times \text{Quantity} = \text{Amount to give}$$

or

$$\frac{15 \text{ gr.}}{5 \text{ gr.}} \times \frac{1 \text{ tablet}}{1} = ? \text{ tablets}$$

$$\frac{15}{5} = 3 \text{ tablets}$$

$$\frac{\text{Dose ordered}}{\text{Dose on hand}} \times \text{Drug form} = \text{Amount to give}$$

or

$$\frac{10 \text{ mg.}}{40 \text{ mg.}} \times 2 \text{ ml.} = \text{Amount to give}$$

$$\frac{20}{40} = 0.5 \text{ ml.}$$

$$\frac{\text{Dose ordered}}{\text{Drug strength on hand}} \times \text{Vehicle} = \text{Amount to give}$$

or

$$\frac{600,000 \text{ U.}}{400,000 \text{ U.}} \times 1 \text{ ml.} = \text{Amount to give}$$

$$\frac{600,000}{400,000} = 1.5 \text{ ml.}$$

Practice Problems:

1. 3/4 gr. = ? mg.

    ANSWER: _____

2. 0.3 Gm. = ? gr.

    ANSWER: _____

3. 0.6 Gm. = ? mg.

    ANSWER: _____

4. 0.2 mg. = ? gr.

    ANSWER: _____

5. 750 mg. = ? Gm.

   ANSWER: _____

6. 0.005 Gm. = ? mg.

   ANSWER: _____

7. 7 1/2 gr. = ? Gm.

   ANSWER: _____

8. 2 fluid drams = ? ml.

   ANSWER: _____

9. 1 1/2 gr. = ? Gm.

   ANSWER: _____

10. 5 gr. = ? mg.

    ANSWER: _____

11. 1 Tbsp. = ? ml.

   ANSWER: _____

12. 0.03 Gm. = ? mg.

   ANSWER: _____

13. 130 lbs. = ? kg.

   ANSWER: _____

14. 2 tsp. = ? ml.

   ANSWER: _____

15. 2 fl. dr. = ? ml.

   ANSWER: _____

16. 20 ml. = ? fl. dr.

   ANSWER: _____

CHAPTER **2**

NONPARENTERAL DRUGS

ORAL DOSAGES

Tablets and Capsules

A general rule for administering ordered dosages of oral medications is that only scored tablets can be divided accurately. Examples of scored tablets can be seen in Figure 1. Usually one gives the ordered dosage using as few tablets as possible.

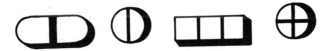

FIGURE 1. Scored tablets.

Enteric-coated tablets and capsules containing powders or timed-release pellets cannot be divided accurately. Therefore it is necessary to look for capsules or enteric-coated tablets of the desired dosage or a dosage that falls within the 10 percent margin of error explained in Chapter 1.

Rarely does a physician order a drug in capsule or tablet form that is not available in the dosage ordered. The most frequent use of a fraction of a tablet occurs in the home when giving medications to a child using the available adult dosage tablet.

Hereinafter, all tablets should be considered as unscored tablets unless otherwise indicated. All examples and practice problems involve the calculation of dosages for adults unless otherwise indicated by age in parentheses.

Before discussing the calculation of oral tablet and capsule doses, it should be noted that this process occasionally is not necessary. The physician may order the number of tablets or capsules to be given. Nurses may safely administer the number of tablets or capsules ordered *if* they are *certain* that the drug is available in one dosage only. For example, "clofibrate one capsule q.i.d.," could be administered safely, since clofibrate comes in 500 mg. capsules only. However, by contrast, an order for "chlorpromazine one tablet t.i.d." cannot be carried out safely because chlorpromazine is available in 10, 50, 100, and 200 mg. tablets.

Examples

PROBLEM 1.   ORDERED: Aspirin 10 gr. q.4h. p.o. p.r.n. for pain.

AVAILABLE: Acetylsalicylic acid (aspirin) 5 gr. tablets.

SOLUTION: FORMULA B

known amounts   *unknown amount*
(available for use) (ordered)   (needed)
dosage:amount = dosage:amount
5 gr.:1 tablet = 10 gr.:x tablet(s)
$5x = 10$
$x = 2$ tablets

ANSWER: Administer 2 aspirin tablets 5 gr. each orally every 4 hours as needed.

Whenever the available medication is labeled in the same unit of measure as the physician's order, only Formula B is needed to solve the problem, as seen above. Both Formula A and Formula B are needed to solve problems in which the available and ordered units of measure differ, as illustrated below. In such instances, note that one may either convert the unit of measure of the tablet available to the same unit of measure as the ordered dosage as in Problem 2, or one may convert the ordered dosage to the same unit of measure as the tablet available as in Problem 3.

PROBLEM 2.   ORDERED: Aspirin 10 gr. q.4h. p.o. p.r.n. for temperature over 102°F.

AVAILABLE: Acetylsalicylic acid (ASA) 0.3 Gm. tablets.

SOLUTION: FORMULA A

known equivalents   *unknown equivalents*
15 gr.:1 Gm. = x gr.:0.3 Gm.
$1x = 4.5$
$x = 4.5$ or 5 gr.,
therefore 0.3 Gm.
equals 5 gr.

FORMULA B

known amounts   unknown amount
(available for use)   (ordered) (needed)
dosage:amount = dosage:amount
5 gr.:1 tablet = 10 gr.:x tablet(s)
5 x = 10
x = 2 tablets

ANSWER: Administer 2 ASA tablets 0.3 Gm. each orally
                       every 4 hours when required for temperature
                       over 102°F.

If the equivalent 16 gr.:1 Gm. had been used above, then 0.3 Gm. would equal 4.8 gr. Actually, whenever a tablet is labeled "0.33 Gm." or "0.3 Gm.," one may assume that this equals 1/3 Gm. or 5 gr. Conversely, one may assume that a tablet labeled "5 gr." equals 0.33 Gm. or 0.3 Gm. Likewise, 10 gr. equals 0.66 Gm. or 0.6 Gm. Remembering this can eliminate much difficulty when doing dosage problems.

PROBLEM 3.   ORDERED: Nembutal 1 1/2 gr. p.o. h.s. p.r.n.

             AVAILABLE: Pentobarbital sodium (Nembutal Sodium) 50
                         and 100 mg. capsules.

SOLUTION: FORMULA A

known equivalents   unknown equivalents
1 gr.:60 mg. = 1 1/2 gr.:x mg.
1 x = 90
x = 90 mg.

or

1 gr.:64 mg. = 1 1/2 gr.:x mg.
1 x = 96
x = 96 mg.

or

15 gr.:1000 mg. = 1 1/2 gr.:x mg.
15 x = 1500
x = 100 mg.

FORMULA B

known amounts   unknown amount
(available for use)   (ordered) (needed)
dosage:amount = dosage:amount
100 mg.:1 capsule = 100 mg.:x capsule(s)
100 x = 100
x = 1 capsule

17

ANSWER: Administer 1 Nembutal 100 mg. capsule orally at hour of sleep (bedtime) when required.

PROBLEM 4. ORDERED: Phenobarbital 15 mg. p.o. q.i.d.

AVAILABLE: Phenobarbital (Luminal) tablets 1/4 gr., 1/2 gr., 1 gr., and 1 1/2 gr.

SOLUTION:

$$60 \text{ mg.}:1 \text{ gr.} = 15 \text{ mg.}:x \text{ gr.}$$
$$60x = 15$$
$$x = 15/1 \div 60$$
$$x = 15/1 \times 1/60$$
$$x = 1/4 \text{ gr.}$$

ANSWER: Administer 1 phenobarbital tablet 1/4 gr. orally 4 times a day.

PROBLEM 5. ORDERED: Digoxin 1/120 gr. p.o. q.d.

AVAILABLE: Digoxin (Lanoxin) tablets 0.25 mg.

SOLUTION:

$$1 \text{ mg.}:1/60 \text{ gr.} = x \text{ mg.}:1/120 \text{ gr.}$$
$$1/60 \, x = 1/120$$
$$x = 1/120 \div 1/60 =$$
$$1/120 \times 60/1 =$$
$$60/120 = 1/2$$
$$x = 0.5 \text{ mg.}$$

$$0.25 \text{ mg.}:1 \text{ tablet} = 0.5 \text{ mg.}:x \text{ tablet(s)}$$
$$0.25 \, x = 0.5$$
$$x = 2 \text{ tablets}$$

ANSWER: Administer 2 Lanoxin tablets 0.25 mg. orally every day.

PROBLEM 6. ORDERED: Phenergan 0.05 Gm. p.o. stat.

AVAILABLE: Promethazine hydrochloride (Phenergan) tablets 12.5 mg. and 25 mg.

SOLUTION:

$$1 \text{ Gm.}:1000 \text{ mg.} = 0.05 \text{ Gm.}:x \text{ mg.}$$
$$1x = 50$$
$$x = 50 \text{ mg.}$$

$$25 \text{ mg.}:1 \text{ tablet} = 50 \text{ mg.}:x \text{ tablet(s)}$$
$$25x = 50$$
$$x = 2 \text{ tablets}$$

ANSWER: Administer 2 Phenergan tablets 25 mg. orally immediately.

Practice Problems:

1. ORDERED: Equanil 0.2 Gm. p.o. q.i.d.

   AVAILABLE: Meprobamate (Miltown, Equanil) scored tablets 400 mg.

   ANSWER: _____

2. ORDERED: Chloromycetin 0.5 Gm. p.o. q.6h.

   AVAILABLE: Chloramphenicol (Chloromycetin) capsules 250 mg.

   ANSWER: _____

3. ORDERED: Prostaphlin 1 Gm. p.o. q.4h.

   AVAILABLE: Oxacillin (Prostaphlin) capsules 250 mg. and 500 mg.

   ANSWER: _____

4. ORDERED: (11-year-old patient) Cortisone 12.5 mg. p.o. q.i.d.

   AVAILABLE: Cortisone acetate scored tablets 5 mg., 10 mg., and 25 mg.

   ANSWER: _____

5. ORDERED: Cortisone 0.025 Gm. p.o. q.i.d.

   AVAILABLE: Cortisone acetate scored tablets 5 mg. and 10 mg.

   ANSWER: _____

19

6. ORDERED: Seconal 1 1/2 gr. p.o. h.s. p.r.n. and may repeat 1 time.

   AVAILABLE: Secobarbital sodium (Seconal sodium) capsules 50 mg.

   ANSWER: _____

7. ORDERED: (4-year-old patient) Sulfadiazine 4 gr. p.o. q.i.d.

   AVAILABLE: Sulfadiazine scored tablets 0.5 Gm.

   ANSWER: _____

8. ORDERED: Sulfadiazine 1.5 Gm. p.o. q.i.d.

   AVAILABLE: Sulfadiazine scored tablets 500 mg.

   ANSWER: _____

9. ORDERED: Neomycin 1 Gm. q.4h. p.o. for 72 hrs. prior to surgery.

   AVAILABLE: Neomycin sulfate tablets 500 mg.

   ANSWER: _____

10. ORDERED: Phenobarbital 1 1/2 gr. p.o. q.i.d.

    AVAILABLE: Phenobarbital sodium tablets 32 mg. and 64 mg.

    ANSWER: _____

11. ORDERED: Atropine 0.5 mg. p.o. q.i.d.

    AVAILABLE: Atropine sulfate tablets 1/200 gr., 1/150 gr., and 1/120 gr.

    ANSWER: _____

12. ORDERED: Dilantin 1 1/2 gr. p.o. t.i.d.

    AVAILABLE: Dilantin sodium capsules 30 mg. and 100 mg. and scored tablets 50 mg.

    ANSWER: _____

DRUGS IN SOLUTION

Drugs Not Requiring Calculations

Some drugs are available in one strength only. They do not have a specific weight measure of drug in a specified volume of solvent. With these drugs, the physician orders the volume amount to be given. No calculation is necessary to determine the amount of the drug to be given. The volume ordered becomes the amount to be administered. Some examples of such orders are as follows:

Alurate elixir ʒi p.o. q.3-4h. p.r.n.
Milk of magnesia ʒi stat.
Lugol's solution 5 drops t.i.d.
Terpin hydrate 5 ml. q.4h. p.r.n. for cough.
Gelusil 30 ml. t.i.d. a.c. and h.s.
Robitussin 5 cc. q.2h. p.r.n. for cough.
SSKI 10 gtts. stat then t.i.d.
Paregoric 5 ml. stat.
Donnatal 5 cc. t.i.d. a.c. and h.s.

One ounce receptacles (Fig. 2) used for administering drugs orally vary but most are marked in drams and milliliters (or cc.) and many also include teaspoon and tablespoon measurements. Therefore, relatively large amounts can be measured quite accurately in one ounce containers.

Other more accurate means should be used to measure less than 5 milliliters and smaller units of measure such as minims and drops. Figure 3 shows an oral syringe used to measure from 0.2 ml. to 10 ml. of solution. A

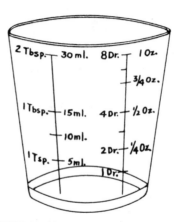

FIGURE 2. One ounce medicine cup.

tuberculin syringe (See Figure 6A, p. 42) can be used to measure up to 16 minims or hundredths of a milliliter.

Drops is an approximate, household unit of measurement; minims is an accurate, apothecaries' unit of measurement. Therefore, one may safely substitute minims for drops, but one should never measure a dosage in drops when minims are ordered. Minim pipettes or syringes may be used to measure minims. Medicine droppers are used to measure drops. The size of drops varies considerably depending upon the viscosity and temperature of the solution, the size of the opening in the dropper, the force with which the solution is expelled, and the angle at which the dropper is held. Holding the dropper at a 45 degree angle is suggested when measuring drugs.

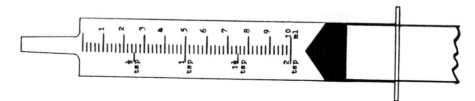

FIGURE 3. Oral syringe.

Some liquid drugs come with a special graduated dropper attached to the lid of the bottle as is illustrated in Figure 4. These are graduated to be used with the specific drug in the bottle to which they are attached.

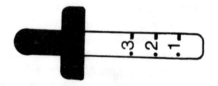

FIGURE 4. Calibrated medicine dropper.

Drugs Requiring Calculations

Solutions for parenteral administration also occasionally are ordered in a volume unit of measure. For example, the physician may order "Bejectal 1 ml. I.M. twice weekly." However, when the physician orders oral or parenteral preparations of drugs in solution, he frequently orders a number of milligrams, grams, or other units of weight measure. Nurses must then convert these to drams, ounces, milliliters, or other units of volume measure in order to administer the prescribed dosage.

Occasionally nurses must use weight to fluid volume measurements to solve dosage or solutions problems. The use of 1 gram equaling 1 milliliter and 1 grain equaling 1 minim are the equivalents most frequently used.

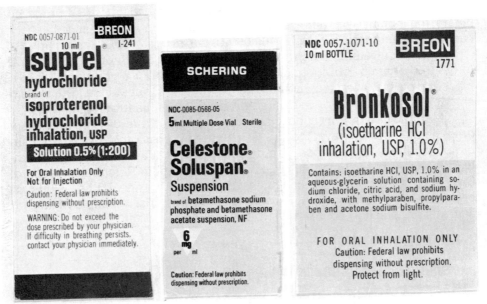

FIGURE 5. Three different labels. (Courtesy of Breon Laboritories, Inc. and the Schering Corporation.)

Labels on drugs in solution may indicate a certain weight measure in a particular volume measure, for example, 500 mg./5 ml. or 10 gr. in 1 dram. Labels on these drugs also may merely state a percentage or a ratio strength of the solutions (Fig. 5).

Whenever the strength of a drug that is available in solution is stated as a ratio or as a percentage strength, the parts are equal parts. A 5% solution therefore may be said to contain 5 Gm. in every 100 ml. It may also be said to contain 5 gr. in every 100 m. because 1 gr. = 1 m. A 1:1000 solution contains 1 gr. in every 1000 m., 1 Gm. in every 1000 ml., 1000 mg. in every 1000 ml., or 1 mg. in every 1 ml. One Gm. of a drug usually does not exactly equal 1 ml., but when administering drugs in solution form we can assume this equality because the pharmacist or pharmaceutical company has weighed, not measured, the drug.

There is 1 Gm. of drug in 1000 ml. of a 1:1000 solution or 1 mg. of drug in 1 ml. of this 1:1000 solution. It does not matter how much of the drug one says is available for administration in the first and second terms of the proportion when calculating the dosage. It is only the strength of the solution available for administration that is important. After determining how much of the solution is needed in order to give the desired dosage, one can determine whether the vial, ampule, or bottle contains enough solution.

Units of measure other than those found in the metric, apothecaries', or household systems may be used to indicate the quantity of a drug either in oral or parenteral solution. Units, abbreviated U., and milliequivalents, abbreviated mEq., are the most commonly used examples. Occasionally such units of measure are used for drugs in tablet or capsule form. Physicians order a quantity of milliequivalents or units. Labels on the drugs indicate the number of milliequivalents or units in a particular volume or capacity measure, for example, 400,000 U. per ml. or 20 mEq. per 15 ml.

A milliequivalent, which is equal to one thousandth of an equivalent, refers to the number of ionic charges of an element or a compound. It is a measure of the chemical combining power of a substance. Potassium chloride (KCl) is an example of a drug ordered in milliequivalents.

Measuring drugs in units means something a little different for every drug measured this way. One U.S.P. insulin unit promotes the metabolism of about 1.5 Gm. of dextrose. The penicillin unit is the equivalent of the antibiotic activity of 0.6 mcg. of U.S.P. Penicillin Sodium Reference Standard. One mg. of this kind of penicillin equals 1,667 units. Other kinds of penicillin have different mg. to units equivalents. For example, 1 mg. of benzathine penicillin equals 1,211 U.S.P. units.

Examples:

PROBLEM 1.   ORDERED: Chloral hydrate liquid 7 1/2 gr. h.s.

                AVAILABLE: Chloral hydrate 10 gr. per fluid dram.

SOLUTION: FORMULA B

$$\begin{array}{cc} known\ amounts & unknown\ amount \\ (available\ for\ use) & (ordered)\quad (needed) \end{array}$$

$$dosage:amount = dosage:amount$$
$$10\ gr.:4\ ml.\ (1\ fl.\ dram) = 7\ 1/2\ gr.:x\ ml.$$
$$10\ x = 30$$
$$x = 3\ ml.$$

ANSWER: Administer 3 ml. chloral hydrate liquid at bedtime.

PROBLEM 2.   ORDERED: Glucose 25 Gm. p.o. t.i.d. today.

                AVAILABLE: Glucose 50% solution.

SOLUTION:	50 Gm.:100 ml. = 25 Gm.:x ml. 50 x = 2500 x = 50 ml.

ANSWER: Administer 50 ml. 50% glucose solution orally 3 times today.

PROBLEM 3. ORDERED: Isotonic sodium chloride (NaCl) 1 Gm. orally-q.6h.

AVAILABLE: Isotonic NaCl (0.9:100) solution.

SOLUTION:

$$0.9 \text{ Gm.}:100 \text{ ml.} = 1 \text{ Gm.}:x \text{ ml.}$$
$$0.9\, x = 100$$
$$x = 100 \div 9/10 =$$
$$100/1 \times 10/9 =$$
$$1000/9 =$$
$$111 \; 1/9 \text{ ml.}$$

ANSWER: Administer approximately 111 1/9 ml. isotonic NaCl solution by mouth every 6 hours.

PROBLEM 4. ORDERED: (5-year-old patient) Sulfadiazine suspension 300 mg. q.i.d.

AVAILABLE: Sulfadiazine suspension 0.25 Gm. per 5 ml.

SOLUTION:

$$1 \text{ Gm.}:1000 \text{ mg.} = x \text{ Gm.}:300 \text{ mg.}$$
$$1000\, x = 300$$
$$x = 0.3 \text{ Gm.}$$

$$0.25 \text{ Gm.}:5 \text{ ml.} = 0.3 \text{ Gm.}:x \text{ ml.}$$
$$0.25\, x = 1.5$$
$$x = 6 \text{ ml.}$$

or

$$1 \text{ Gm.}:1000 \text{ mg.} = 0.25 \text{ Gm.}:x \text{ mg.}$$
$$1\, x = 250$$
$$x = 250 \text{ mg.}$$

$$250 \text{ mg.}:5 \text{ ml.} = 300 \text{ mg.}:x \text{ ml.}$$
$$250\, x = 1500$$
$$x = 6 \text{ ml.}$$

ANSWER: Administer 6 ml. sulfadiazine suspension 4 times a day.

PROBLEM 5.   ORDERED: (18-month-old patient) Potassium gluconate 10 mEq. p.o. q.i.d.

              AVAILABLE: Kaon elixir (potassium gluconate) 20 mEq./ 15 ml.

SOLUTION: 20 mEq.:15 ml. = 10 mEq.:x ml.
                                        20 x = 150
                                            x = 7.5 ml.

ANSWER: Administer 7.5 ml. Kaon elixir orally every 6 hours.

PROBLEM 6.   ORDERED: (4-year-old patient) V-Cillin K 300,000 U. q.4h. p.o.

              AVAILABLE: Potassium phenoxymethyl penicillin (V-Cillin K) 125 mg. or 200,000 U. per 5 ml.

SOLUTION: 200,000 U.:5 ml. = 300,000 U.:x ml.
                                      200,000 x = 1,500,000
                                            x = 7.5 ml.

ANSWER: Administer 7.5 ml. V-Cillin K every 4 hours by mouth.

Practice Problems:

1. ORDERED: Paregoric 5 ml. stat.

    AVAILABLE: Paregoric ℥ii.

    ANSWER: _____

2. ORDERED: (3-year-old patient) V-Cillin K 0.25 Gm. p.o. q.6h.

    AVAILABLE: Potassium phenoxymethyl penicillin (V-Cillin K) 125 mg. or 200,000 U./5 ml.

    ANSWER: _____

3. ORDERED: Kaochlor 30 mEq. p.o. q.d.

    AVAILABLE: Kaochlor 10% (20 mEq. potassium per 15 ml.)

    ANSWER: _____

4. ORDERED: Mycostatin oral suspension 500,000 U. t.i.d.

    AVAILABLE: Nystatin (Mycostatin) oral suspension 100,000 units per ml.

    ANSWER: _____

5. ORDERED: (2-year-old child) Amoxicillin 50 mg. p.o. q.i.d.

    AVAILABLE: Larotid (Amoxicillin) 50 mg./ml. pediatric drops and 125 or 250 mg./5 ml. oral suspensions.

    ANSWER: _____

6. ORDERED: Paregoric and milk of bismuth ʒi $\overline{aa}$ t.i.d.

    AVAILABLE: Paregoric and milk of bismuth ʒi $\overline{aa}$ in one 2 oz. bottle.

    ANSWER: _____

7. ORDERED: (20-month-old baby) Ephedrine liquid 3 mg. q.4h. p.r.n.

    AVAILABLE: Ephedrine sulfate 1/8 gr. per 5 cc.

    ANSWER: $\frac{1}{60}$ gr : 1mg. : x 3mg

    $x = \frac{1}{20}$ gr

    1/8 gr : 5ml :: 1/20 x

8. ORDERED: (3-year-old patient) Digoxin 0.02 mg. p.o. q.d.

   AVAILABLE: Lanoxin Elixir Pediatric (Digoxin) 0.05 mg./cc. with dropper marked in tenths of a ml.

   ANSWER: _____

9. ORDERED: (8-year-old patient) Gantrisin suspension 0.4 Gm. q.4h

   AVAILABLE: Sulfisoxazole (Gantrisin) suspension 100 mg. per ml.

   ANSWER: _____

10. ORDERED: Elixir terpin hydrate with codeine 1/8 gr. for cough.

    AVAILABLE: Terpin hydrate and codeine elixir 2 mg. per ml.

    ANSWER: _____

11. ORDERED: (13-year-old patient) Ilotycin suspension 400 mg. q.6h.

    AVAILABLE: Erythromycin (Ilotycin) suspension 0.2 Gm. per 5 cc.

    ANSWER: _____

12. ORDERED: Kaon elixir 20 mEq. t.i.d.

    AVAILABLE: Potassium gluconate (Kaon) 20 mEq. per 15 ml.

    ANSWER: _____

PREPARING ORAL SOLUTIONS

Occasionally nurses need to prepare oral solutions from crystals or powder as in Problem 1. Sometimes they may need to prepare children's dosages from adult dosage tablets if the drug is not readily available in the pediatric liquid or tablet form and the tablet available cannot be divided accurately by breaking it. If the tablet is soluble in water, it can be crushed and dissolved in a specified amount of water. Then the ordered dosage can be accurately measured in a syringe. See Problem 2.

PROBLEM 1.   ORDERED: 250 ml. 1/2 isotonic saline p.o. q.h. × 4.

AVAILABLE: Table salt and home cooking measures.

It should be remembered that isotonic saline is a 0.9% strength solution and that 1 gram = 1 milliliter. Since the oral solution is ordered for four doses (×4), it would be easier to prepare all four doses at one time, or 1000 ml. (4 × 250 ml.).

SOLUTION: FORMULA B

known amounts   *unknown amount*
(to be prepared for use)   (to be prepared for use)
(strength to be prepared)   (totals in container)

$$dosage{:}amount = dosage{:}amount$$
$$0.45 \text{ Gm.}{:}100 \text{ ml.} = x \text{ Gm.}{:}1000 \text{ ml.}$$
$$100\,x = 450$$
$$x = 4.5 \text{ Gm.}$$

ANSWER: Add 1 tsp. salt to a qt. of water if preparing the entire amount at one time or 1/4 tsp. salt to a glass of water if preparing 250 ml. at a time.

PROBLEM 2.   ORDERED: (1-year-old child) Sudafed 10 mg. p.o. q.6h.

AVAILABLE: Pseudoephedrine HCl (Sudafed) 60 mg. tablets.

The nurse can arbitrarily choose the amount of solution in which to give the ordered dose of the drug. In this example the nurse chose to use 4 ml.

SOLUTION: FORMULA B

known amounts   *unknown amount*
(to be prepared for use)   (to be prepared for use)
(strength to be prepared)   (totals in container)

$$dosage{:}amount = dosage{:}amount$$
$$10 \text{ mg.}{:}4 \text{ ml.} = 60 \text{ mg.}{:}x \text{ ml.}$$
$$10\,x = 240$$
$$x = 24 \text{ ml.}$$

Therefore, if one wants to give 10 mg. in 4 ml., dissolve one of the 60 mg. Sudafed tablets in 24 ml. of solution and give 4 ml. orally every 6 hours.

or

The nurse can choose the amount of solution in which to dissolve the tablet. In this example the nurse chose to use 30 ml.

known amounts (to be prepared for use) (totals in container)	*unknown amount* (to be prepared for use) (strength to be prepared)

$$dosage{:}amount = dosage{:}amount$$
$$60 \text{ mg.}{:}30 \text{ ml.} = 10 \text{ mg.}{:}x \text{ ml.}$$
$$60\,x = 300$$
$$x = 5 \text{ ml.}$$

ANSWER:

Therefore, if one chooses to dissolve one of the 60 mg. Sudafed tablets in 30 ml. of water, do so, and give 5 ml. orally every 6 hours.

or

The nurse can determine the fraction of the tablet that will be needed.

$$60 \text{ mg.}{:}1 \text{ tablet} = 10 \text{ mg.}{:}x \text{ tablet}$$
$$60\,x = 10$$
$$x = 1/6 \text{ tablet}$$

In this instance the denominator can be interpreted as the total volume in which to dissolve the tablet (for example 6 ml.). The numerator can be interpreted as the dose to be given (in this example, 1 ml.).

Practice Problems:

1. ORDERED: 250 ml. 5% dextrose p.o. t.i.d.

    AVAILABLE: Dextrose powder.

    ANSWER: _____

2. ORDERED: (1-year-old child) Phenobarbital 12 mg. p.o. q.12h.

    AVAILABLE: Phenobarbital sodium tablets 30, 60, or 100 mg. each.

    ANSWER: _____

3. ORDERED: (1-year-old child) Phenobarbital 15 mg. p.o. q.8h.

    AVAILABLE: Luminal sodium (phenobarbital sodium) 60, 125, 200, or 300 mg. powder in 2 ml. ampules.

    ANSWER: _____

4. ORDERED: (1-year-old child) Dimetane 1.25 mg. p.o. q.i.d.

    AVAILABLE: Brompheniramine maleate (Dimetane) 4 mg. tablets.

    ANSWER: _____

PREPARING TOPICAL SOLUTIONS

This section is included more as a reference than for actual use since solutions used topically usually are available from stock supplies, or they are prepared by the pharmacy in the strength desired. Occasionally, however, nurses in small hospitals or in community health settings may need to prepare solutions for hospital use or instruct patients how to prepare solutions for topical use in their homes. Also, the nurse may need to know how to prepare solutions for oral use, such as a 1:3 solution of hydrogen peroxide as a mouth wash.

When preparing solutions for topical or oral use, one is changing the percentage or ratio strength of the drug to a weaker strength, or to the strength ordered or desired for use. One or two variations of Formula B can be used to solve all types of solution problems, which include:

1. Preparing solutions from tablets, powders, or crystals (always 100% strength)
2. Preparing solutions from stock solutions
   a. From 100% strength solutions
   b. From less than 100% strength solutions

Tablets, Powders, or Crystals

Though the drugs added to the solvent often increase the total volume slightly, the amount of increase is too small to make any appreciable difference when preparing large amounts of solution. Also, the displacement by the drug may be 0.5 ml. or 2 ml., for example, and one may be using a 1-liter pitcher, with a mark for every 50 ml., to measure the solvent. It is impossible to measure accurately enough to account for these small displacement amounts. Therefore, the amount of displacement by the drug is not considered when the drug is in tablet, crystal, or powder form.

Because in actual practice the containers available for measurement of large volumes are calibrated for every 50 or 100 ml., for example, accurate measurement of the stock drug or solution to within a fraction of a milliliter or even to within a few milliliters is not possible. It may be necessary to measure small amounts of solute in a 1 ounce container, for example, and to measure the solvent in another much larger container.

Examples:

PROBLEM 1. ORDERED: Warm saturated boric acid solution soaks of left foot 20 min. stat. (Assume one needs 1 gal. of this solution.)

AVAILABLE: Boric acid crystals.

SOLUTION: A 5% boric acid solution is a saturated one.

$$known\ amounts \qquad\qquad unknown\ amount$$
$$\text{(to be prepared for use)} \quad \text{(to be prepared for use)}$$
$$\text{(strength to be prepared)} \quad \text{(totals in container)}$$
$$dosage{:}amount = dosage{:}amount$$
$$5\ Gm.{:}100\ ml. = x\ Gm.\ (ml.){:}4000\ ml.$$
$$100\ x = 20{,}000$$
$$x = 200\ Gm.\ (ml.)$$

ANSWER: Add 200 ml. boric acid crystals to 1 gal. warm water.

Weighing 200 Gm. of boric acid crystals would be more accurate than measuring 200 ml. of the drug, but scales are not available in clinical areas or in homes. When preparing solutions for topical use, attaining the exact ordered strength is not as important as when giving oral or parenteral dosages. Therefore, in this instance one may safely substitute ml. for Gm. when measuring powders or crystals.

PROBLEM 2. ORDERED: N.S. enema p.r.n. (One decides to prepare 2 qts. of this solution.)

AVAILABLE: Table salt.

Normal saline is a 5.8% strength solution. Normal saline solutions are rarely used because they are physiologically hypertonic rather than isotonic. Physiologically isotonic saline is a 0.9% strength solution. However, when dealing with drugs in solution and parenteral fluids the abbreviation "N.S." is used for normal saline and the strength intended is 0.9%, the strength of isotonic saline. When ordered by the physician, 1/2 N.S. would be 0.45% strength and 1/4 N.S. would be 0.2% strength.

SOLUTION:

$$known\ amounts \qquad unknown\ amount$$
$$dosage:amount = dosage:amount$$
$$0.9\ Gm.:100\ ml. = x\ Gm.\ (ml.):2000\ ml.$$
$$100\ x = 1800$$
$$x = 18\ Gm.\ (ml.)$$

ANSWER:

Add 18 ml. table salt to 2 qts. of tap water at the appropriate temperature. (Because of the heavy molecular weight of sodium chloride, 2 tsp. salt per qt. of water may be used when preparing isotonic saline solutions.)

PROBLEM 3.   ORDERED:

1:8000 potassium permanganate ($KMnO_4$) compresses to right lower leg 20 min. q.i.d. (Assume one needs 1 qt. of this solution.)

AVAILABLE: $KMnO_4$ tablets 300 mg. (5 gr.)

SOLUTION:

$$1\ Gm.:8000\ ml. = x\ Gm.:1000\ ml.$$
$$8000\ x = 1000$$
$$x = 1/8\ Gm. = 2\ gr.$$

Potassium permanganate tablets cannot be divided. Therefore, prepare the ordered strength of solution by using 1 of the 5 gr. tablets, as shown below.

SOLUTION:

$$1\ Gm.:8000\ ml. = 0.3\ Gm.:x\ ml.$$
$$1\ x = 8000 \times 0.3$$
$$x = 2400\ ml.$$

or

$$1\ mg.:8\ ml. = 300\ mg.:x\ ml.$$
$$1\ x = 8 \times 300$$
$$x = 2400\ ml.$$

ANSWER:

Dissolve 1 of the 300 mg. (5 gr. or 1/3 Gm.) $KMnO_4$ tablets in 2400 ml. sterile water. (Use sterile water as the solvent because the patient has an open lesion on his leg.)

A potassium permanganate solution may be used for bactericidal or bacteriostatic action because it is an oxidizing agent. Exposure to light or heat before use causes loss of oxygen which makes the solution ineffective as an antiseptic or germicidal solution. Therefore, prepared solutions should not be heated and they should be stored in a dark, cool place. Also, potassium permanganate stains fabrics and skin. The stains are difficult to remove.

PROBLEM 4. ORDERED: Sterile warm 2% boric acid compresses continuously today. (One wants to dissolve all of the drug.)

AVAILABLE: One oz. of boric acid crystals.

SOLUTION:

$$2 \text{ Gm.}:100 \text{ ml.} = 30 \text{ Gm. (ml.)}:x \text{ ml.}$$
$$2x = 3000$$
$$x = 1500 \text{ ml.}$$

ANSWER: Dissolve the 1 oz. of boric acid crystals in 1 1/2 qts. sterile water.

Practice Problems:

1. ORDERED: N.S. enema stat. (Assume that one needs 1 qt. of this solution.)

AVAILABLE: Sodium chloride crystals.

ANSWER: _____

2. ORDERED: Irrigate both eyes with 3% sodium bicarbonate solution stat. (One wants to prepare 2 qts. solution.)

AVAILABLE: Sodium bicarbonate.

ANSWER: _____

3. ORDERED: 1000 ml. mercuric chloride 1:1000 for disinfection purpose.

   AVAILABLE: Mercury bichloride tablets 0.5 Gm. and 0.12 Gm.

   ANSWER: _____

4. ORDERED: Paint feet with 1:1000 gentian violet b.i.d. q.d. (Prepare 1 oz.)

   AVAILABLE: Gentian violet tablets 10 mg., 15 mg., and 30 mg.

   ANSWER: _____

5. ORDERED: 1:10,000 $KMnO_4$ soaks of both legs 20 min. t.i.d. (One needs 1 gal. of solution.)

   AVAILABLE: $KMnO_4$ tablets 300 mg. (5 gr.).

   ANSWER: _____

6. ORDERED: 1:8000 potassium permanganate ($KMnO_4$) soaks to left foot 30 min. b.i.d. (One needs at least 1 qt. solution.)

   AVAILABLE: $KMnO_4$ tablets 300 mg. (5 gr.).

   ANSWER: _____

7. **ORDERED:** Warm saturated boric acid solution compresses to lesions on right leg 20 minutes q.i.d. (One needs 1 qt. solution each treatment.)

    AVAILABLE: Boric acid crystals and 1000 ml. bottles of sterile water.

    ANSWER: _____

8. **ORDERED:** Rinse mouth with 2% sodium perborate q.i.d. (Prepare 100 ml. each time.)

    AVAILABLE: Sodium perborate powder.

    ANSWER: _____

Stock Solutions

As stated earlier, occasionally nurses may need to solve problems involving the dilution of stock solutions to make weaker solutions. The strength of the solution to be prepared for use may be stated as a ratio, for example, 1:4, or as a percentage strength such as 2%. The strength of the stock solution available also may be expressed as a ratio or as a percentage strength, either 100% or less than 100%.

Remember, to properly represent the strength of a percent solution, a 5% solution can be said to contain 5 grams of drug in every 100 milliliters of solution, or a 5% solution also can be said to contain 5 grains of drug in every 100 minims of solution. To properly represent the strength of a ratio solution, a 1:1000 solution can be said to contain 1 gram of drug in every 1000 milliliters of solution (1 Gm. in 1000 ml. or 1000 mg. in 1000 ml. or 1 mg. in 1 ml.), or 1 grain of drug in every 1000 minims of solution. Examples are shown below.

PROBLEM 1. ORDERED: Dilute hydrogen peroxide 1:4 and use as mouthwash q.i.d. (One needs 1 oz. for each treatment.)

AVAILABLE: Hydrogen peroxide (3%).

SOLUTION:

known amounts   *unknown amount*

(to be prepared for use)   (to be prepared for use)

(strength to be prepared)   (totals in container)

dosage:amount = *dosage:amount*

$1:4 = x$ ml.:32 ml.

$4x = 32$

$x = 8$ ml.

ANSWER:
Use 8 ml. of 3% hydrogen peroxide and 24 ml. water. (There are 20% hydrogen peroxide preparations but these are not for medicinal use. The 3% hydrogen peroxide is rarely used as a mouthwash without further dilution of either 1:3 or 1:4.)

PROBLEM 2. ORDERED:
Hydrogen peroxide 1:3 mouthwash t.i.d. (One needs 2 oz. for each treatment.)

AVAILABLE:
Hydrogen peroxide (3%).

SOLUTION:

$1:3 = x$ ml.:60 ml.

$3x = 60$

$x = 20$ ml.

ANSWER:
Use 20 ml. of 3% hydrogen peroxide and 40 ml. water.

When determining how to prepare solutions from stock solutions of less than 100% strength, two variations of Formula B must be used. The first step is to determine the amount of drug needed to prepare the desired strength and amount of solution. The second step is to determine the amount of stock solution needed in order to obtain this amount of drug. See examples below.

PROBLEM 3. ORDERED:
30% alcohol cooling sponge stat. (Assume one needs 2 qts. solution.)

AVAILABLE:
70% isopropyl alcohol.

SOLUTION: Step 1. Amount of drug needed

known amounts   *unknown amount*

(to be prepared for use)   (to be prepared for use)

(strength to be prepared)   (totals in container)

dosage:amount = *dosage:amount*

30 Gm.:100 ml. = x Gm.:2000 ml.

$100x = 60,000$

$x = 600$ Gm.

Step. 2. Amount of solution needed

	known amounts	unknown amount
	(available for use)	(needed to be used)
	(strength available)	(totals in solution)

$$dosage:amount = dosage:amount$$
$$70 \text{ Gm.}:100 \text{ ml.} = 600 \text{ Gm.}:x \text{ ml.}$$
$$70 \, x = 60{,}000$$
$$x = 857 \, 1/7 \text{ ml.}$$

ANSWER: Use 857 1/7 ml. 70% alcohol and 1142 6/7 ml.
tap water. (These amounts do not have to be
measured this accurately, of course.)

PROBLEM 4. ORDERED: 2% Lysol solution for disinfecting excreta.
(One needs 3 qts. solution.)

AVAILABLE: Saponated cresol (Lysol) solution 1:2.

SOLUTION: Step 1.

$$2 \text{ Gm.}:100 \text{ ml.} = x \text{ Gm.}:3000 \text{ ml.}$$
$$100 \, x = 6000$$
$$x = 60 \text{ Gm.}$$

Step 2.

$$1 \text{ Gm.}:2 \text{ ml.} = 60 \text{ Gm. (ml.)}:x \text{ ml.}$$
$$1 \, x = 120$$
$$x = 120 \text{ ml.}$$

ANSWER: ✓ Add 2880 ml. water to 120 ml. Lysol 1:2.

Practice Problems

1. ORDERED: Sponge with 25% alcohol stat. (One needs 2 quarts of
this solution.)

AVAILABLE: One pint bottles of 70% isopropyl alcohol.

ANSWER: _____

2. ORDERED: 4 oz. 2.5% dextrose solution p.o. q.3h.

AVAILABLE: 50 ml. ampules 50% dextrose and 500 ml. and 1000 ml.
bottles of 5% and 10% dextrose.

ANSWER: _____

3. **ORDERED:** 1:3 alcohol sponge p.r.n. (One decides to use 1 pint of alcohol.)

   AVAILABLE: One pint bottles of 70% isopropyl alcohol.

   ANSWER: _____

4. **ORDERED:** 1:50 Lysol solution for disinfecting excreta. (One needs 1 gal. of the solution.)

   AVAILABLE: 1 gallon bottles of 50% Lysol.

   ANSWER: _____ water

5. **ORDERED:** Apply 1:1000 Adrenalin to left nostril stat.

   AVAILABLE: Epinephrine solution 1:100.

   ANSWER: _____

6. **ORDERED:** Hydrogen peroxide (3%) diluted 1:3 as mouthwash q.i.d. (One needs 1 oz. each time.)

   AVAILABLE: Hydrogen peroxide (3%) in 1 pt. bottles.

   ANSWER: _____

7. ORDERED: Soak both feet in Dakin's solution (0.5%) 15 min. t.i.d.
                  (One needs 2 qts. for each treatment.)

    AVAILABLE: Sodium hypochlorite solution 5%.

    ANSWER: _____

8. ORDERED: Irrigate left eye c̄ 2% boric acid solution q.i.d. (Assume
                  one wants to prepare 500 ml. sterile solution.)

    AVAILABLE: Sterile 5% boric acid solution.

    ANSWER: _____

OTHER NONPARENTERAL DRUGS

Suppositories are another common vehicle for administering medications.
Suppositories can be administered via the rectum, vagina, or urethra. They
are melted by the body temperature and absorption occurs locally. They
are usually ordered in the doses which are available and no calculations
are necessary.

There are also topical ointments that rely on local absorption. No
calculations are necessary for this type of medication; however, specific
directions should be read thoroughly and followed carefully.

CHAPTER 3
PARENTERAL DRUGS

DRUGS IN SOLUTION

Problems involving the parenteral administration of drugs are solved in exactly the same way as the oral solutions problems in Chapter 2. However, all answers are in minims and/or milliliters because this is how syringes are calibrated. Drug strengths may be shown in any of the following ways:

gr./ml.
mg./ml.
Gm./ml.
mEq./ml.
U./ml.
percent (Gms./100 ml.)
ratio (1:1000 or 1 Gm./1000 ml.)

The more common syringes that are available are illustrated in Figure 6.

Examples:

PROBLEM 1. ORDERED: Streptomycin 500 mg. b.i.d. I.M.

AVAILABLE: Streptomycin sulfate 1 Gm. in 2 ml.

SOLUTION: FORMULA A

known equivalents   *unknown equivalents*
1 Gm.:1000 mg. = x Gm.:500 mg.
1000 x = 500
x = 0.5 Gm.

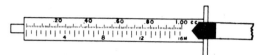

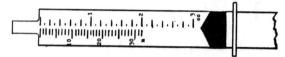

A. Tuberculin syringe.

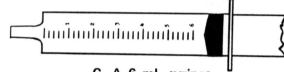

B. A 3 ml. syringe.

C. A 6 ml. syringe.

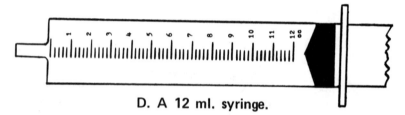

D. A 12 ml. syringe.

FIGURE 6. Syringes.

FORMULA B

known amounts   unknown amount
(available for use)   (ordered)   (needed)
dosage:*amount* = *dosage*:*amount*
1 Gm.:2 ml. = 0.5 Gm.:*x* ml.
1 *x* = 1
x = 1 ml.

ANSWER: Administer 1 ml. streptomycin sulfate (1 Gm. in 2 ml.) intramuscularly twice daily.

PROBLEM 2.   ORDERED: Codeine 30 mg. s.c. q.4h. p.r.n. for pain.

AVAILABLE: 20 ml. vial codeine sulfate labeled "1 gr. in 1 ml."

SOLUTION:

60 mg.:1 gr. = 30 mg.:*x* gr.
60 *x* = 30
x = 1/2 gr.

1 gr.:1 ml. = 1/2 gr.:*x* ml.
1 *x* = 1/2
x = 0.5 ml.

ANSWER:	Administer 0.5 ml. codeine sulfate subcuta-neously every 4 hours when required for pain.

PROBLEM 3. ORDERED: Adrenalin 0.4 mg. "H" q.3h. p.r.n. for asthma.

AVAILABLE: 1 ml. ampules epinephrine (Adrenalin) 1:1000 (1 Gm.:1000 ml. or 1 gr.:1000 m.).

SOLUTION: 1 Gm.:1000 ml. or
1000 mg.:1000 ml. or 1 mg.:1 ml.

$$1 \text{ mg.:1 ml.} = 0.4 \text{ mg.:} x \text{ ml.}$$
$$1x = 0.4$$
$$x = 0.4 \text{ ml.}$$

ANSWER: Administer 0.4 ml. epinephrine 1:1000 sub-cutaneously or intramuscularly every 3 hours as needed.

PROBLEM 4. ORDERED: Levo-Dromoran 1.5 mg. s.c. q.6h. p.r.n. for pain.

AVAILABLE: Levorphanol tartrate (Levo-Dromoran) 1 ml. ampules labeled "2 mg. per ml."

SOLUTION:
$$2 \text{ mg.:16 m. (1 ml.)} = 1.5 \text{ mg.:} x \text{ m.}$$
$$2x = 24$$
$$x = 12 \text{ m.}$$

ANSWER: Administer 12 m. Levo-Dromoran subcutane-ously every 6 hours as needed for pain.

Note that 16 m. was used as the equivalent of 1 ml.; therefore, 2 ml. equals 32 m. Whenever drugs are given with a hypodermic or tuberculin syringe, use 16 m. = 1 ml. rather than 15 m. = 1 ml. when calculating the amount to be given. This gives a more accurate answer because these syringes are calibrated either with 16 m. per ml. or 16 plus m. per ml., not with 15 m. per ml. Hypodermic syringes are calibrated in tenths of ml. also. To give 1.25 ml., fill the syringe to the point one-half way between 1.2 and 1.3 ml. To give 1.33 ml. fill the syringe to the point as nearly one-third of the way between 1.3 and 1.4 ml. as possible. Tuberculin syringes are calibrated in hundredths of ml. as well as in minims. When measuring small amounts of parenteral solutions, for example, 2 m. or 0.125 ml., use of a tuberculin syringe is desirable.

PROBLEM 5. ORDERED: Procaine penicillin 400,000 U. I.M. b.i.d.

AVAILABLE: 10 ml. vial procaine penicillin G 300,000 U. per ml.

SOLUTION:	
	300,000 U.:1 ml. = 400,000 U.:x ml.
	300,000 x = 400,000
	3 x = 4
	x = 1.33 ml.

ANSWER: Administer 1.33 ml. procaine penicillin G intramuscularly twice a day.

PROBLEM 6. ORDERED: Calcium gluconate 1 Gm. I.V. stat.

AVAILABLE: 10 ml. ampule calcium gluconate 10% (10 Gm.:100 ml.)

SOLUTION:

$$10 \text{ Gm.}:100 \text{ ml.} = 1 \text{ Gm.}:x \text{ ml.}$$
$$10 x = 100$$
$$x = 10 \text{ ml.}$$

ANSWER: Administer 10 ml. of 10% calcium gluconate intravenously immediately. (Nurse will prepare; physician will administer.)

PROBLEM 7. ORDERED: (5 kg. infant) Epinephrine s.c. stat according to the pediatric emergency room's basic dosage guideline of "0.01 ml./kg./dose of the 1:1000 solution (1 mg./ml.) for small children and infants."

AVAILABLE: 1 ml. ampules of epinephrine 1:1000.

SOLUTION:

$$0.01 \text{ ml.}:1 \text{ kg.} = x \text{ ml.}:5 \text{ kg.}$$
$$1 x = 0.05 \text{ ml. } (0.05 \text{ mg.})$$

Even with a 1 ml. tuberculin syringe, it is difficult to measure very accurately such a small amount of solution. Further dilution of the 1:1000 strength solution allows for the administration of a larger volume for greater accuracy of measurement. Therefore, one could add 1 ml. of epinephrine 1:1000 to a vial containing 4 ml. of sterile distilled water, making a strength of 1:5000 (1 mg./5 ml.). A greater dilution than this requires that an unnecessarily large volume be given subcutaneously to this small infant.

SOLUTION:

$$1 \text{ mg.}:5 \text{ ml.} = 0.05 \text{ mg.}:x \text{ ml.}$$
$$1 x = 0.25 \text{ ml.}$$

ANSWER: Administer 0.25 ml. of the epinephrine diluted to a 1:5000 strength subcutaneously immediately.

By using the 1:5000 strength solution, the 10% margin of error gives one a range of 0.225 ml. to 0.275 ml. to be measured instead of a range of 0.045 ml. to 0.055 ml. if the 1:1000 strength were used.

Practice Problems:

1. ORDERED: Heparin 100 mg. s.c. q.8h.

    AVAILABLE: A 2 ml. vial of sodium heparin injection 40,000 units per ml. (1 mg. = 100 units.)

    ANSWER: _____

2. ORDERED: Cedilanid-D 0.6 mg. I.M. q.d.

    AVAILABLE: 2 ml. and 4 ml. ampules of deslanoside (Cedilanid-D) containing 0.4 mg. and 0.8 mg. respectively.

    ANSWER: _____

3. ORDERED: (1-year-old patient) Cedilanid-D 0.025 mg. I.M. stat.

    AVAILABLE: 2 ml. and 4 ml. ampules deslanoside (Cedilanid-D) containing 0.4 mg. and 0.8 mg. respectively.

    ANSWER: _____

4. ORDERED: AquaMephyton 20 mg. I.M. stat.

    AVAILABLE: 1 ml. ampules of phytonadione solution (AquaMephyton) 2 or 10 mg. per ml.

    ANSWER: _____

5. ORDERED: (8 1/4 pound infant) Epinephrine s.c. stat. using standing order of "0.01 mg./kg./dose."

    AVAILABLE: 1 ml. ampules of epinephrine 1:1000.

    ANSWER: _____

6. ORDERED: Hypaque 50 mg. intradermally at 9 a.m. tomorrow.

    AVAILABLE: 1 cc. ampules 50% Hypaque sodium solution.

    ANSWER: _____

7. ORDERED: Reserpine 5 mg. I.M. stat.

    AVAILABLE: 2 ml. ampules containing Serpasil (reserpine) 2.5 mg.
                  per ml.

    ANSWER: _____

8. ORDERED: Procaine penicillin 500,000 U. I.M. b.i.d.

    AVAILABLE: 10 cc. vial Wycillin (procaine penicillin G in aqueous
                  suspension) 300,000 units per cc.

    ANSWER: _____

9. ORDERED: Adrenalin 0.5 mg. "H" q.3h. p.r.n. for asthma.

    AVAILABLE: 30 ml. vial epinephrine (Adrenalin) 1:2000.

    ANSWER: _____

10. ORDERED: Tigan 200 mg. I.M. stat. then 100 mg. q.6h. p.r.n. nausea.

    AVAILABLE: 20 ml. vial and 2 ml. ampules trimethobenzamide hydro-
                  chloride (Tigan HCl) 100 mg. per ml.

    ANSWER: _____

11. ORDERED: Aminophylline 0.5 Gm. I.M. q.i.d. p.r.n. for asthma.

    AVAILABLE: 2 cc. ampule containing Aminophylline 500 mg. (7 1/2 gr.).

    ANSWER: _____

12. ORDERED: (2-year-old patient) M.S. 2 mg. "H" pre-op at 10 a.m.

    AVAILABLE: 30 ml. vial morphine sulfate 16.2 mg. (1/4 gr.) per ml.

    ANSWER: _____

DRUGS REQUIRING RECONSTITUTION

Some penicillins, antibiotics, and other drugs to be given parenterally are stored in crystal or powder form in sterile vials or ampules. Before these drugs are administered they must be dissolved in a desirable diluent or solvent, usually sterile isotonic saline or sterile distilled water labeled "for injection." A sterile syringe is used to withdraw the diluent from one vial and to add it to the vial or ampule containing the drug in its dry form. After the drug has been dissolved in this diluent, the correct volume can be administered to the patient.

Please note: Multidose vials of sterile isotonic saline or sterile water for injection contain a bacteriostatic preservative which has been discovered to cause seizures in neonates (up to 1 month, at least), whether these diluents are used to reconstitute drugs for intramuscular or intravenous use. Single dose vials of these solutions to be used as diluent do not contain a preservative and may be used.

If the entire amount of drug in the vial is to be given at one time, add enough diluent to dissolve the drug, usually at least 1 to 2 ml. The amount needed to dissolve the drug varies with the type and amount of drug in the vial or ampule. Directions for dissolving drugs for parenteral administration usually can be found on the vial, on the box containing the vial, or on a pamphlet in the accompanying box. In some manner, these directions usually indicate the amount of volume that the drug itself occupies *after* it is in solution. For example, directions may say that adding 1.2 ml. sterile distilled water yields 2 ml. of reconstituted solution. In other words, although the drug itself occupies considerably less space when in solution than when in the dry form, this particular drug still displaces 0.8 ml. in volume measurement. In order to get a 5 ml. total amount of solution in this particular vial, add 4.2 ml. diluent. If one added 5 ml. diluent, there would be 5.8 ml. in the vial.

Figures 7A and 7B show that powders or crystals occupy a greater volume when in dry form than after they have been dissolved in a diluent.

Figures 7B and 7C show that when enough diluent to dissolve the drug has been added, the drug will occupy the same volume of space no matter how much more diluent is added. The drug will be dispersed throughout the total amount of solution.

In Figure 7B each ml. of reconstituted drug solution contains one-fifth of the 1 Gm. of drug, or 200 mg. In Figure 7C each ml. of reconstituted drug solution contains one-tenth of the 1 Gm. of drug, or 100 mg.

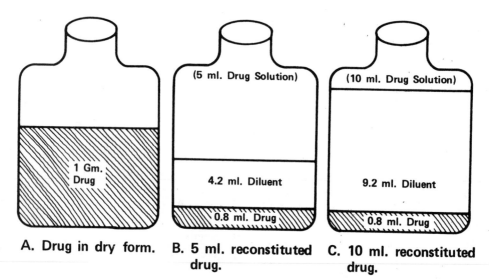

A. Drug in dry form.   B. 5 ml. reconstituted   C. 10 ml. reconstituted
                            drug.   drug.

FIGURE 7. Displacement by 1 Gm. of drug.

Figure 8A shows one way that directions for reconstitution may be given. Adding 18 ml. of diluent yields a solution of penicillin G containing 250,000 U./ml. and a total of 20 ml. containing the total 5,000,000 U. of drug.

$$250,000 \text{ U.}:1 \text{ ml.} = 5,000,000 \text{ U.}:x \text{ ml.}$$
$$250,000\, x = 5,000,000$$
$$x = 20 \text{ ml.}$$

The drug therefore occupies 2 ml. of that 20 ml. volume. If 3 ml. of diluent were added, each ml. of the prepared penicillin G solution would contain 1,000,000 U./ml. There would be 5 ml. total solution, 2 ml. of which would be the drug.

$$1,000,000 \text{ U.}:1 \text{ ml.} = 5,000,000 \text{ U.}:x \text{ ml.}$$
$$1,000,000\, x = 5,000,000$$
$$x = 5 \text{ ml.}$$

Directions in Figure 8B indicate that adding 1 ml. diluent will result in a solution of ampicillin containing 250 mg./ml. In such instances the total amount of prepared solution will be slightly more than 1 ml. Therefore, there must be a little more than 250 mg. of ampicillin in the vial.

$$250 \text{ mg.} : 1 \text{ ml.} = x \text{ mg.} : 1 + \text{ml.}$$
$$x = 250^+ \text{ mg.}$$

Figure 8C shows one of many variations of ready-to-mix vials in which the diluent is provided in the vial but separate from the drug in dry powder or crystal form. These vials provide a mechanism for releasing the diluent from the upper part of the vial into the lower part of the vial containing the drug. In this instance, addition of the diluent in the vial will yield approximately 3.0 ml. of prepared cefazolin solution containing 330 mg./ml. Therefore, the vial contains 1 Gm. of cefazolin.

$$330 \text{ mg.} : 1 \text{ ml.} = x \text{ mg.} : 3 \text{ ml.}$$
$$x = 990 \text{ mg. or } 1 \text{ Gm.}$$

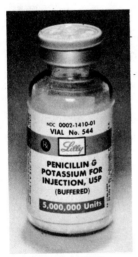

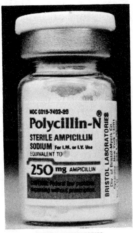

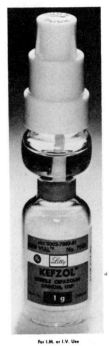

CAUTION—Federal (U.S.A.) law prohibits dispensing without prescription.
Prior to Reconstitution: Store at 59° to 86°F (15° to 30°C).
Usual Adult Dose—Intramuscularly, 400,000 units 4 times a day. Intravenously, 10,000,000 units a day. See literature. Sterile solution may be kept in refrigerator for 7 days without significant loss of potency.
Contains sodium citrate - citric acid buffer.

PREPARATION OF SOLUTION

Add diluent	Concentration of Solution
18 ml	250,000 Units/ml
8 ml	500,000 Units/ml
3 ml	1,000,000 Units/ml

A.

BRISTOL LABORATORIES
Div. of Bristol-Myers Co.
Syracuse, New York 13201
For I.M. use, add 1 ml diluent (read accompanying circular).
Resulting solution contains 250 mg ampicillin per ml.
   Use solution within 1 hour.
This vial contains ampicillin sodium equivalent to 250 mg ampicillin.
Usual Dosage: Adults—250 to 500 mg I.M. q. 6h.
READ ACCOMPANYING CIRCULAR for detailed indications, I.M. or I.V. dosage and precautions.
© 1977 Bristol Laboratories
   740220DRL-14

Lot

Exp. Date

B.

For I.M. or I.V. Use
Dosage—See Literature

To prepare solution, turn top of cap clockwise and push down to dislodge center plug. Remove cap.
   SHAKE WELL TO DISSOLVE
Diluent contains Water for Injection, with 0.9% Benzyl Alcohol.

Withdraw entire contents to provide 1 g dose.

Provides an approximate volume of 3.0 ml (330 mg per ml).
After reconstitution—Store in a refrigerator and use within 96 hours. If kept at room temperature, use within 24 hours.

Protect from Light
YC 0954 AMX
Eli Lilly & Co., Indpls., IN 46285, U.S.A.
Exp. Date/Control No.

C.

FIGURE 8. Drugs requiring reconstitution. (Courtesy of Eli Lilly and Company and Brestol Laboratories.)

Currently, very few drugs are given intramuscularly. Whenever possible, most drugs to be given parenterally are given intravenously. This is primarily because a therapeutic level of drug in the blood stream can be attained and maintained more effectively via the intravenous route. Absorption of drugs from the muscle is quite unpredictable and dependent upon many variables. Also, as will be seen in this chapter, the amount that would be given intramuscularly is often quite large.

However, it should be noted that all problems in this section of this chapter are the same as the first step in the administration of drugs intravenously; that is, (1) reconstitute the drug if necessary, and (2) calculate the correct amount of reconstituted solution to use in order to give the ordered dosage of the drug.

Although the directions for reconstitution of drugs given here may seem confusing, all directions are those actually found for these drugs which are currently being given. As will be seen, one can only conclude that there are occasional inconsistencies in the directions, or that the amount of drug in the vial is slightly more than the label claims; therefore, the directions are correct.

Sometimes the vial contains more than one ordered dose. Whenever only a portion of the reconstituted drug is used, the vial should be properly labeled so that the remaining drug may be given later. Because the ordered dosage is often available in 1 ml., it is a safety precaution to label vials with the dosage per ml., for example, "200,000 U./ml.," or "0.5 Gm./ml.," even though the ordered dosage may be less or more than the amount of drug in 1 ml.

Most drugs should be refrigerated after reconstitution. Drug pamphlets tell how long the drug remains stable at room temperature or refrigerated. Therefore, place the date and time on the label. Many agencies require nurses to put their names on the labels of drugs that they reconstitute.

All parenteral solutions problems can be solved with the proportion Formula B, starting with the amounts known to be available for or prepared for use. It may be necessary to use Formula A first if the ordered and available dosages are not in the same unit of measurement.

Examples:

PROBLEM 1.   ORDERED: Penicillin G 2,000,000 U. I.M. q.3h.

AVAILABLE: Penicillin G (crystalline penicillin G sodium) vial containing 5,000,000 units in dry form.

DIRECTIONS:

Diluent	Concentration
23 ml.	200,000 U./ml.
18 ml.	250,000 U./ml.
8 ml.	500,000 U./ml.
3 ml.	1,000,000 U./ml.

SOLUTION:

known amounts   unknown amount

(available for use)   (ordered)   (needed)

$$1,000,000 \text{ U.}:1 \text{ ml.} = 2,000,000 \text{ U.}:x \text{ ml.}$$
$$1,000,000\ x = 2,000,000$$
$$x = 2 \text{ ml.}$$

ANSWER: Add 3 ml. diluent to the vial and give 2 ml. I.M. q.3h.

There will be 2 1/2 doses in this vial.

$$2,000,000 \text{ U.}:1 \text{ dose} = 5,000,000 \text{ U.}:x \text{ dose(s)}$$
$$2,000,000\ x = 5,000,000$$
$$x = 2\ 1/2 \text{ doses}$$

If there are 1,000,000 U./ml. when 3 ml. diluent is added the drug displacement is 2 ml.

known amounts   unknown amount

(prepared for use)   (totals in vial)

$$dosage{:}amount = dosage{:}amount$$
$$1,000,000 \text{ U.}:1 \text{ ml.} = 5,000,000 \text{ U.}:x \text{ ml.}$$
$$1,000,000\ x = 5,000,000$$
$$x = 5 \text{ ml.}$$
$$\underline{-3 \text{ ml/diluent}}$$
$$2 \text{ ml. drug}$$
$$\text{displacement}$$

Using the same calculations it would be found that following these directions yields a consistent amount of drug displacement. This is not always so, as will be shown later.

Diluent	Concentration	Total amount drug solution	Amount of drug displacement
23 ml.	200,000 U./ml.	25 ml.	2 ml.
18 ml.	250,000 U./ml.	20 ml.	2 ml.
8 ml.	500,000 U./ml.	10 ml.	2 ml.
3 ml.	1,000,000 U./ml.	5 ml.	2 ml.

Sometimes the directions for reconstitution of a drug do not include a dosage exactly the same as the amount ordered, as in Problem 2 below.

PROBLEM 2. ORDERED: Penicillin G 300,000 U. I.M. q.2h.

             AVAILABLE: Same as in Problem 1 above.

             DIRECTIONS: Same as in Problem 1 above.

| SOLUTION: | Select one or more concentrations in the directions which are closest to the ordered dosage, for example, 250,000 U./ml. or 500,000 U./ml. |

known amounts   *unknown amount*
(prepared)   (ordered)
dosage:amount   *dosage:amount*

250,000 U.:1 ml. = 300,000 U.:x ml.
250,000 x = 300,000
x = 1.2 ml.

or

500,000 U.:1 ml. = 300,000 U.:x ml.
500,000 x = 300,000
x = 0.6 ml.

| ANSWER: | Two actions would be reasonable: 1) Add 18 ml. diluent to this vial and give 1.2 ml. I.M. q.2h., or, 2) add 8 ml. diluent and give 0.6 ml. I.M. q.2h. |

PROBLEM 3.   **ORDERED:**   Penicillin G Potassium 300,000 U. I.M. q.2h.

AVAILABLE: Penicillin G Potassium (crystalline penicillin G potassium) vial containing 1,000,000 units in dry form.

DIRECTIONS:

Label	Diluent	U./ml.
1,000,000	9.6 ml.	100,000
1,000,000	4.6 ml.	200,000
1,000,000	3.6 ml.	250,000

SOLUTION:

200,000 U.:1 ml. = 300,000 U.:x ml.
200,000 x = 300,000
x = 1.5 ml.

or

250,000 U.:1 ml. = 300,000 U.:x ml.
250,000 x = 300,000
x = 1.2 ml.

| ANSWER: | Two actions would be acceptable, although action 2 results in a smaller volume to be given to the patient: 1) Add 4.6 ml. diluent to |

52

this vial and give 1.5 ml. I.M. q.2h., or, 2) Add 3.6 ml. diluent and give 1.2 ml. I.M. q.2h.

In either instance, since there are 1,000,000 units in this vial and 300,000 units are ordered, there are 3 1/3 doses in this vial.

$$300,000 \text{ U.:1 dose} = 1,000,000 \text{ U.:} x \text{ doses}$$
$$300,000 \, x = 1,000,000$$
$$x = 3 \, 1/3 \text{ doses}$$

PROBLEM 4. ORDERED: (1-year-old infant) Mefoxin 200 mg. I.M. q.4h.

AVAILABLE: Mefoxin (cefoxidan sodium) vial containing 1 Gm. of dry powder.

DIRECTIONS:

Strength	Diluent	Approximate withdrawal	Approximate concentration
1 Gm.	2 ml.ˣ	2.5 ml.	400 mg./ml.
2 Gm.	4 ml.ᵻ	5.0 ml.	400 mg./ml.

SOLUTION:

$$400 \text{ mg.:1 ml.} = 200 \text{ mg.:} x \text{ ml.}$$
$$400 \, x = 200$$
$$x = 0.5 \text{ ml.}$$

ANSWER: Add 2 ml. diluent to the 1 Gm. vial and give 0.5 ml. I.M. q.4h. or add 4 ml. to the 2 Gm. vial and give 0.5 ml. I.M. q.4h. There would be 5 doses in the 1 Gm. vial and 10 doses in the 2 Gm. vial.

All of the above problems have been examples of consistent displacement directions. Problem 5 is an example of inconsistent displacement directions.

PROBLEM 5. ORDERED: Staphcillin 1 Gm. I.M. q.6h.

AVAILABLE: Staphcillin (methicillin sodium) 1 Gm., 4 Gm., and 6 Gm. vials.

DIRECTIONS: To get a concentration of approximately 500 mg./ml.:
Add 1.5 ml. diluent to 1 Gm. vial
Add 5.7 ml. diluent to 4 Gm. vial
Add 8.6 ml. diluent to 6 Gm. vial

SOLUTION:
(prepared)   (ordered)
$$500 \text{ mg.:1 ml.} = 1000 \text{ mg. (1 Gm.):} x \text{ ml.}$$
$$500 \, x = 1000$$
$$x = 2 \text{ ml.}$$

ANSWER: Add 1.5 ml. diluent to 1 Gm. vial and give
                              2 ml. I.M. q.6h.

In Problem 5, above, if there are 500 mg./ml. in the 1 Gm. vial after 1.5 ml. of diluent is added, there should be 2 ml. of reconstituted solution. If so, the drug displacement would be 0.5 ml.

Diluent	Vial	Strength	Volume	Displacement
1.5 ml.	1 Gm.	500 mg./ml.	2 ml.	0.5 ml.
5.7 ml.	4 Gm.	500 mg./ml.	8 ml.	2.3 ml.
8.6 ml.	6 Gm.	500 mg./ml.	12 ml.	3.4 ml.

If there are 500 mg./ml. in the 4 Gm. vial after 5.7 ml. of diluent is added there should be 8 ml. of reconstituted solution. If so, the calculated drug displacement would be 2.3 ml., not 2 ml., or four times as much displacement for 4 Gm. as for 1 Gm., as one would expect.

If there are 500 mg./ml. in the 6 Gm. vial after 8.6 ml. of diluent is added, there would be 12 ml. If so, the drug displacement would be 3.4 ml., not 3 ml. or six times the displacement for 1 Gm. of drug.

One can only hope that the amounts of drugs in these three vials are not exactly 1, 4, and 6 Gm., but that the exact amount of drug has been altered to make the directions for reconstitution correct. If not, the directions are incorrect. One has no way of knowing which, if any, of the directions are correct. One can only follow the directions for the most appropriate concentration and hope that the margin of error, if any, does not exceed 10%. Other examples of apparent discrepancies in reconstitution directions will be included in the practice and review problems.

PROBLEM 6.   ORDERED: Keflin 0.5 Gm. I.M. q.4h.

             AVAILABLE: Keflin (cephalothin sodium) 1 Gm. vial in dry
                           form.

             DIRECTIONS: Dilute 1 Gm. in minimum of 4 ml. diluent.

SOLUTION: Such directions do not give any information
                           about drug displacement or the concentra-
                           tion of the reconstituted drug.

ANSWER: One can only add 4 ml. of diluent, withdraw
                           the entire amount of reconstituted solution,
                           and give one-half of the entire amount. (The
                           0.5 Gm. ordered is one-half of the 1 Gm. in
                           the vial.) Label vial 0.5 Gm. in exact remain-
                           ing amount as measured.

Practice Problems:

1. ORDERED: Cephadyl 600 mg. I.M. q.4h.

   AVAILABLE: Cephadyl (cephapirin sodium) in dry form in 500 mg., 1 Gm., and 2 Gm. vials.

   DIRECTIONS: Reconstitute 500 mg. and 1 Gm. vials with 1 ml. and 2 ml. respectively to get 500 mg./1.2 ml.

   ANSWER: _____

2. ORDERED: Polycillin-N 200 mg. I.M. q.4h.

   AVAILABLE: Polycillin-N (ampicillin sodium) in dry form in 125 mg., 250 mg., 500 mg., 1 Gm., and 2 Gm. vials.

   DIRECTIONS:

Label claim	Amount diluent	Withdrawal volume	Concentration of mg./ml.
125 mg.	1.2 ml.	1 ml.	125 mg.
250 mg.	1.0 ml.	1 ml.	250 mg.
500 mg.	1.8 ml.	2 ml.	250 mg.
1 Gm.	3.5 ml.	4 ml.	250 mg.
2 Gm.	6.8 ml.	8 ml.	250 mg.

   ANSWER: _____

3. ORDERED: Geopen 1 Gm. I.M. q.6h.

   AVAILABLE: Geopen (carbenicillin disodium) in dry form in 1 Gm., 2 Gm., and 5 Gm. vials.

   DIRECTIONS: Add minimum of 2 ml. diluent to a 1 Gm. vial.

Diluent to 1 Gm. vial	Volume for 1 Gm. dose	(Calculated displacement)
2.0 ml.	2.5 ml.	0.5 ml./Gm.
2.5 ml.	3.0 ml.	0.5 ml./Gm.
3.6 ml.	4.0 ml.	0.4 ml./Gm.

Add minimum of 4 ml. diluent to 2 Gm. vial.

Diluent to 2 Gm. vial	Volume for 1 Gm. dose	(Calculated displacement)
4.0 ml.	2.5 ml.	0.5 ml./Gm.
5.0 ml.	3.0 ml.	0.5 ml./Gm.
7.2 ml.	4.0 ml.	0.4 ml./Gm.

The inclusion of "calculated displacements" above and hereafter are by the authors, not the pharmaceutical companies.

   ANSWER: _____

4. ORDERED: Geopen 1.5 Gm. I.M. q.6h.

   AVAILABLE: Same as in Problem 3 above.

   DIRECTIONS: Same as in Problem 3 above.

   ANSWER: _____

5. ORDERED: Prostaphlin 750 mg. I.M. q.4h.

   AVAILABLE: Prostaphlin (oxacillin sodium) in dry form in 250 mg.,
                   500 mg., 1 Gm., 2 Gm., and 4 Gm. vials.

   DIRECTIONS: To obtain a solution containing 250 mg. of drug in 1.5
                   ml. of solution:

Vial	Diluent	(Calculated displacement per 250 mg.)
250 mg.	1.4 ml.	0.1 ml.
500 mg.	2.7 ml.	0.15 ml.
1 Gm.	5.7 ml.	0.075 ml.
2 Gm.	11.5 ml.	0.0625 ml.
4 Gm.	23.0 ml.	0.0625 ml.

   ANSWER: _____

6. ORDERED: Coly-Mycin 100 mg. I.M. stat and q.12h.

   AVAILABLE: Coly-Mycin (colistimethate sodium) in dry form in
                   150 mg. vials.

   DIRECTIONS: Adding 2 ml. diluent yields 75 mg./ml.

   ANSWER: _____

7. **ORDERED:**   Claforan 1 Gm. I.M. q.8h.

   AVAILABLE: Claforan (cefotaxime sodium) in dry form in 500 mg., 1 Gm., and 2 Gm. vials.

   DIRECTIONS:

Strength	Amount diluent	Approximate withdrawal volume (ml.)	Approximate concentration of mg./ml.
500 mg.	2 ml.	2.2 ml.	230
1 Gm.	3 ml.	3.4 ml.	300
2 Gm.	5 ml.	6.0 ml.	330

   ANSWER: _____

8. **ORDERED:**   (3-month-old infant) Moxam 250 mg. I.M. q.8h.

   AVAILABLE: Moxam (moxalactam disodium) dry powder in 1 Gm. and 2 Gm. vials.

   DIRECTIONS: Dilute every Gm. with 3 ml. diluent.

   ANSWER: _____

9. **ORDERED:**   Mandol 750 mg. I.M. q.6h.

   AVAILABLE: Mandol (cefamandole nafate) dry powder in 500 mg., 1 Gm., and 2 Gm. vials.

   DIRECTIONS: Dilute each Gm. with 3 ml. diluent.

   ANSWER: _____

10. ORDERED: (1-year-old infant) Omnipen-N 100 mg. I.M. q.6h.

    AVAILABLE: Omnipen-N (ampicillin sodium) in dry form in 125 mg.,
                    250 mg., 500 mg., 1 Gm., and 2 Gm. vials.

    DIRECTIONS: Add 1 ml. to 125 mg. vial to get 125 mg./ml.
                    Add 0.9 ml. to 250 mg. vial to get 250 mg./ml.

Label claim	Amount diluent	Withdrawal volume	Concentration in mg./ml.	(Calculated displacement)
500 mg.	1.8 ml.	2.0 ml.	250 mg.	0.10 ml./250 mg.
1 Gm.	3.4 ml.	4.0 ml.	250 mg.	0.15 ml./250 mg.
2 Gm.	6.8 ml.	8.0 ml.	250 mg.	0.15 ml./250 mg.

    ANSWER: _____

11. ORDERED: Pipracil 1 Gm. I.M. q.4h.

    AVAILABLE: Pipracil (piperacillin sodium) in dry form in 2 Gm., 3
                    Gm., and 4 Gm. vials.

    DIRECTIONS: No more than 2 Gm. per injection site. Reconstitute
                    every Gm. with a minimum of 2 ml. of diluent.

Volume of diluent for following vial sizes			Volume to be withdrawn for a 1 Gm. dose
2 Gm.	3 Gm.	4 Gm.	2.5 ml.
4.0 ml.	6.0 ml.	7.8 ml.	

    ANSWER: _____

12. ORDERED: Kefzol 1 Gm. I.M. q.6h.

    AVAILABLE: Kefzol (cefazolin sodium) dry powder in 250 mg., 500
                    mg., and 1 Gm. vials.

    DIRECTIONS:

Vial Size	Diluent	Approximate volume	Approximate Average concentration
250 mg.	2 ml.	2.0 ml.	125 mg./ml.
500 mg.	2 ml.	2.2 ml.	225 mg./ml.
1 Gm.	2 ml.	3.0 ml.	330 mg./ml.

    ANSWER: _____

INSULIN

This section, like the section on Preparing Solutions for Topical Use, is presented more for information than for practice in calculations of insulin dosages.

The 1980s marked the change to only 100 U./ml. insulin in the United States. Insulin of 40 U./ml. is still manufactured but is under study for the feasibility of its continued use. Most hospitals and pharmacies stock only 100 U./ml. insulin.

The past 25 years have seen many improvements in insulin with respect to purity, concentrations, peak time, dosage requirements and methods of administration.

Huminsulin should be available for use in the United States during the 1980s. Huminsulin is the product of the synthesis of human insulin using bacteria genetically altered by recombinant DNA technology. It can be used by persons with sensitivities to the currently used beef and pork insulins.

The types of insulin (rapid-acting, intermediate-acting and long-acting) and injection techniques are changing rapidly. It is not within the scope of this book to discuss these in detail. Type of insulin and the dosage amounts of insulin are determined by the physician for each patient.

The most common method of administration of insulin is by the sub-cutaneous route, using the standard insulin syringe which is now available in 100 U./ml. and 50 U./0.5 ml. (See Figs. 9A and 9B.)

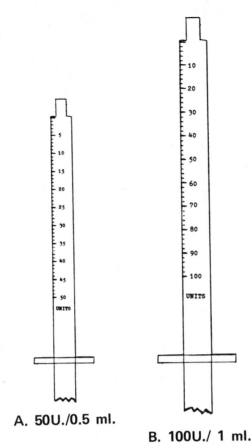

A. 50U./0.5 ml.

B. 100U./ 1 ml.

FIGURE 9. Insulin syringes.

Since insulin is available in 100 U./ml., the amount of insulin ordered is the amount to be measured into the 50 U. or 100 U. syringe. For example, if 26 units of insulin is ordered it would be drawn into the 50 U. syringe as illustrated below in Figure 10A. If 64 units of insulin is ordered it would be drawn into the 100 U. syringe as illustrated in Figure 10B. The 26-unit dosage could be given with the 100 U. syringe but the 64-unit dosage could not be given with the 50 U. syringe.

Different methods of administration currently are being studied. They include a closed-loop insulin infusion intravenously using a computer to act as a feedback mechanism to regulate the insulin flow; an open-loop system that can be used intravenously or subcutaneously with the patient regulating the insulin input; and a continuous subcutaneous insulin infusion system that may be attached externally or implanted with the patient controlling the input of insulin.

One of the newest, more conventional methods of administering insulin is the Medi-Jector® syringe produced by Derata Corporation (Fig. 11.). This syringe is pictured approximately one-half its actual size. The syringe may appear to be large and cumbersome, but it has several advantages over the conventional syringe. The insulin vial is attached directly to the

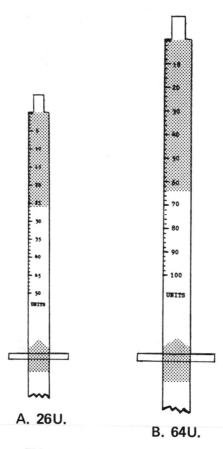

A. 26U.

B. 64U.

FIGURE 10. Insulin dosages.

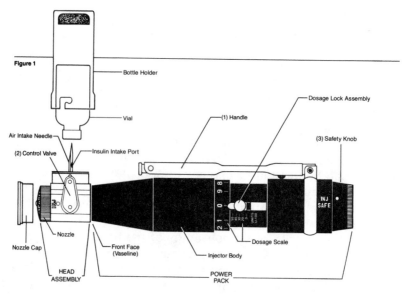

FIGURE 11. Derata Medi-Jector® syringe. (Courtesy of Derata Corporation.)

syringe one time and remains there until the last dose is given. This cuts down on the number of chances for contamination. The insulin dosage is preset and remains constant until changed. This cuts down on the number of times that errors in dosage might be made and also allows the diabetic with diminished vision to safely administer a preset dosage.

Perhaps one of the most important advantages is the way the medication enters the skin when administered by this jet pressure-propelled syringe (Fig. 12.). With this type of dispersion of medication into the subcutaneous tissue, the absorption should be faster and the local tissue trama lessened.

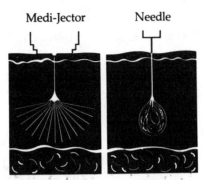

Medi-Jector   Needle

FIGURE 12. Comparative dispersion pattern. (Courtesy of Derata Corporation.)

One might use a hypodermic or a tuberculin syringe when insulin syringes are not available, or when the amount of insulin to be given exceeds the capacity of the available insulin syringes. With the use of these syringes, the ordered insulin dosages must be calculated in minims or in tenths or hundredths of milliliters, as shown below.

Examples:

PROBLEM 1.   ORDERED: Regular insulin 80 U. deep s.c. stat.

AVAILABLE: Regular insulin U. 100 and no insulin syringe.

SOLUTION: FORMULA B

known amounts   unknown amount
(available for use)   (ordered)   (needed)
dosage:amount   dosage:amount
100 U.:1 ml. = 80 U.:x ml.
100 x = 80
x = 0.8 ml.

or

100 U.:16 m. = 80 U.:xm.
100 x = 1280
x = 12.8 m.

ANSWER: Use a tuberculin syringe and give 0.8 ml. or
                                 12.8 m. insulin immediately, deep subcuta-
                                 neously. (These measurements should be at
                                 the same point on the syringe.)

Tuberculin syringes have a 1 ml. volume. They have two scales: one is
calibrated in minims, the other in hundredths of a ml. When small volumes
of insulin are to be given, the correct dosage can be determined more accurately by using a tuberculin syringe than by using a hypodermic syringe.

PROBLEM 2. ORDERED: Regular insulin 40 units a.c. q.a.m.

            AVAILABLE: Regular insulin U. 100 and no insulin syringe.

SOLUTION: 100 U.:1 ml. = 40 U.:x ml.
                                          100 x = 40
                                             x = 0.4 ml.

                                              or

                                     100 U.:16 m. = 40 U.:x m.
                                          100 x = 640
                                             x = 6.4 m.

ANSWER: Use a tuberculin syringe and give 0.4 ml.
                                 or 6.4 m. of insulin before breakfast every
                                 morning.

Sometimes two kinds of insulin are given at the same time, as in the
following problem.

PROBLEM 3. ORDERED: Regular insulin 16 units c̄ N.P.H. insulin 30
                                 units a.c. q .a.m.

            AVAILABLE: Regular insulin U. 100 and N.P.H. insulin U.
                                 100, and no insulin syringes.

SOLUTION: 100 U.:1 ml. = 16 U.:x ml.
                                          100 x = 16
                                             x = 0.16 ml. regular insulin

                                     100 U.:1 ml. = 40 U.:x ml.
                                          100 x = 40
                                             x = 0.4 ml. N.P.H. insulin

ANSWER: Total solution needed is 0.56 ml. (0.16 ml.
                                 regular insulin plus 0.4 ml. N.P.H. insulin).
                                 Using a tuberculin syringe measure 0.16 ml.
                                 of regular insulin into the syringe and then

fill to the 0.56 mark with N.P.H. insulin and administer every morning before breakfast.

PROBLEM 4. ORDERED: Regular insulin 16 U. with N.P.H. insulin 30 U. a.c. every a.m.

AVAILABLE: Regular insulin 100 U. N.P.H. insulin 100 U. and a 50 U. and a 100 U. insulin syringe.

ANSWER: A total measurement of 46 U. (16 U. of regular and 30 U. of N.P.H.) is needed, therefore, a 50 U. insulin syringe can be used. Inject 30 U. of air into the N.P.H. insulin bottle and remove syringe. Inject 16 U. of air into the regular insulin vial and withdraw 16 U. of regular insulin. Put syringe into the N.P.H. insulin vial and withdraw insulin to the 46 U. mark (30 U.). Administer as ordered.

Practice Problems:

1. ORDERED: Regular insulin 10 units 20 min. a.c. t.i.d.

AVAILABLE: Iletin (regular) insulin 100 U. and no insulin syringes.

ANSWER: _____

2. ORDERED: P.Z.I. insulin 18 units 4 p.m. q.d.

AVAILABLE: Protamine zinc insulin (P.Z.I.) 50 U. and 100 U. scale insulin syringe and hypodermic and tuberculin syringes.

ANSWER: _____

3. ORDERED: Regular insulin v̄ units 20 min. a.c. t.i.d.

   AVAILABLE: Crystalline zinc (regular) insulin 100 U. and no insulin
                 syringes.

   ANSWER: _____

4. ORDERED: N.P.H. insulin 24 units 1 hr. a.c. breakfast q.d.

   AVAILABLE: Isophane insulin suspension (N.P.H.) 100 U. and 0.5 ml.
                 (50 units) U. 100 and 1 ml. (100 units) U. 100 scale insu-
                 lin syringes.

   ANSWER: _____

5. ORDERED: N.P.H. insulin 45 units and regular insulin 24 units 1 hr.
                 a.c. breakfast tomorrow.

   AVAILABLE: Isophane insulin suspension (N.P.H.) 100 U. and Iletin
                 (regular) insulin 100 U. and a 100 U. insulin syringe.

   ANSWER: _____

6. ORDERED: Lente insulin 46 units 1 hr. a.c. breakfast q.d.

   AVAILABLE: Insulin zinc suspension (lente) 100 U. and a 100 U. insu-
                 lin syringe and hypodermic and tuberculin syringes.

   ANSWER: _____

7. ORDERED: Ultralente insulin U. 65 1 hr. a.c. breakfast tomorrow.

   AVAILABLE: Insulin zinc suspension, extended (Ultralente Iletin) U. 100 insulin, hypodermic, and tuberculin syringes.

   ANSWER: _____

8. ORDERED: Semilente insulin 18 U. 1/2 hr. a.c. breakfast q.d.

   AVAILABLE: Insulin zinc suspension, prompt (Semilente Iletin) U. 100 and no insulin syringes.

   ANSWER: _____

9. ORDERED: Ultralente insulin 46 units 1 hr. a.c. breakfast q.d.

   AVAILABLE: Ultralente insulin U. 100 and 0.5 ml. and 1 ml. U. 100 scale insulin syringes.

   ANSWER: _____

INTRAVENOUS FLUIDS AND MEDICATIONS

This is one of the most important sections of this book because: (1) currently, many drugs are given intravenously (I.V.), and (2) an error in giving drugs intravenously is more serious than an error with drugs given orally or by injection, where there is more time to take corrective action.

The equipment and supplies used to administer I.V. fluids and/or medications are so numerous that a complete explanation of these is beyond the scope of this book. However, some of these will be illustrated in a discussion designed to proceed from simpler to more complex I.V. solutions and drug problems.

When administering fluids intravenously, nurses often must calculate and regulate the drops per minute in order to give a certain amount in the ordered period of time. The administration sets made by various manufacturers (Fig. 13) are constructed to yield varying numbers of drops per milliliter. This information is found on the box containing the set. Examples are as follows:

10 drops/ml.—Travenol
15 drops/ml.—Abbott
20 drops/ml.—Cutter
60 drops/ml.—Microdrip administration sets made by various companies

Ratio and proportion (or variations of Formula B) can be used to calculate the regulation of intravenous fluids as shown in the third and fourth solutions to Problems 1 and 2 below. However, most nurses seem to pre-

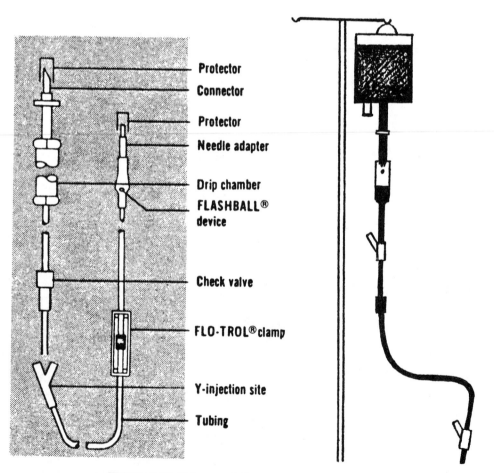

Protector
Connector
Protector
Needle adapter
Drip chamber
FLASHBALL® device
Check valve
FLO-TROL® clamp
Y-injection site
Tubing

FIGURE 13. Primary I.V. administration set.

fer to use the method shown below when calculating the drops per minute that an I.V. should flow. The steps in calculating drops per minute are to determine:

A. ml./hr.
$$\frac{\text{Total ml. fluid to be given}}{\text{hrs. to be run}} = \text{Desired ml./hr.}$$

B. gtts./hr.
$$\text{Desired ml./hr.} \times \text{gtts./ml.} = \text{Desired gtts./hr.}$$

C. gtts./min.
$$\frac{\text{Desired gtts./hr.}}{60 \text{ min.}} = \text{Desired gtts./min.}$$

Steps B and C can easily be reversed as follows:

A. ml./hr.
$$\frac{\text{Total ml. fluid to be given}}{\text{hrs. to be run}} = \text{Desired ml./hr.}$$

B. ml./min.
$$\frac{\text{Desired ml./hr.}}{60 \text{ min.}} = \text{Desired ml./min.}$$

C. gtts./min.
$$\text{Desired ml./min.} \times \text{gtts./ml.} = \text{Desired gtts./min.}$$

Examples:

The simplest type of I.V. problem involves the continuous administration of I.V. solutions, with or without medications added to the I.V. solution bag or bottle (Fig. 13). The connector is inserted into the primary solution container. The roller clamp ("FLO-TROL clamp" in Figure 13) is used to adjust the number of drops per minute.

PROBLEM 1.   ORDERED: Give 1000 ml. 5% dextrose in water (D-5-W) I.V. in 2 hrs.

AVAILABLE: Abbott administration set.

SOLUTION:
A.   1000 ml. ÷ 2 hrs. = 500 ml./hr.
B.   500 ml. × 15 gtts. = 7500 gtts./hr.
C.   7500 gtts. ÷ 60 min. = 125 gtts./min.

or

A.   1000 ml. ÷ 2 hrs. = 500 ml./hr.
B.   500 ml. ÷ 60 min. = 8 1/3 ml./min.
C.   8 1/3 ml. × 15 gtts. = 125 gtts./min.

or

69

A.   1000 ml.:2 hrs. = x ml.:1 hr.
$$2x = 1000$$
$$x = 500 \text{ ml./hr.}$$

B.   1 ml.:15 gtts. = 500 ml.:x gtts.
$$1x = 7500$$
$$x = 7500 \text{ gtts./hr.}$$

C.   7500 gtts.:60 min. = x gtts.:1 min.
$$60x = 7500$$
$$x = 125 \text{ gtts./min.}$$

or

A.   1000 ml.:2 hrs. = x ml.:1 hr.
$$2x = 1000$$
$$x = 500 \text{ ml./hr.}$$

B.   500 ml.:60 min. = x ml.:1 min.
$$60x = 500$$
$$x = 8\ 1/3 \text{ ml./min.}$$

C.   1 ml.:15 gtts. = 8 1/3 ml.:x gtts.
$$1x = 25/3 \times 15/1 = 125$$
$$x = 125 \text{ gtts./min.}$$

ANSWER: Regulate I.V. to flow at 125 drops per minute initially.

PROBLEM 2. ORDERED: Give 2000 ml. D-5-W q.d. by continuous drip.

              AVAILABLE: Travenol administration set.

SOLUTION: A.   2000 ml. ÷ 24 hrs. = 83 1/3 ml./hr.
              B.   83 1/3 ml. × 10 gtts. = 833 1/3 gtts./hr.
              C. 833 1/3 gtts. ÷ 60 min. = 13.88 1/3 or 14 gtts./min.

or

              A.   2000 ml. ÷ 24 hrs. = 83 1/3 ml./hr.
              B.   83 1/3 ml. ÷ 60 min. = 25/18 ml./min.
              C.   25/18 ml. × 10 gtts. = 250/18 = 13 8/9 or 14 gtts./min.

or

A.   2000 ml.:24 hrs. = x ml.:1 hr.
$$24x = 2000$$
$$x = 83\ 1/3 \text{ ml./hr.}$$

B.   1 ml.:10 gtts. = 83 1/3 ml.:x gtts.
$$1 x = 833\ 1/3$$
$$x = 833\ 1/3\ \text{gtts./hr.}$$

C.   833 1/3 gtts.:60 min. = x gtts.:1 min.
$$60 x = 833\ 1/3$$
$$x = 13.88\ 1/3\ \text{or } 14\ \text{gtts./min.}$$

or

A.   2000 ml.:24 hrs. = x ml.:1 hr.
$$24 x = 2000$$
$$x = 83\ 1/3\ \text{ml./hr.}$$

B.   83 1/3 ml.:60 min. = x ml.:1 min.
$$60 x = 83\ 1/3$$
$$x = 1\ 7/18\ \text{ml./min.}$$

C.   1 ml.:10 gtts. = 1 7/18 ml.:x gtts.
$$1 x = 13\ 8/9$$
$$x = 13\ 8/9\ \text{or } 14\ \text{gtts./min.}$$

ANSWER: Regulate to flow at 14 drops per minute initially.

Nurses should check the rate of flow of intravenous fluids at least every 30 minutes for patients whose I.V. sets are not connected to automatic flow control devices and every hour otherwise. It is not enough to count the drops per minute at these intervals because the fluid may have been running faster or slower than it should have been sometime during this interval. Therefore, every time one checks, refigure the rate of flow needed after determining how much fluid is left and in what period of time it is to be administered. See example below.

PROBLEM 3. ORDERED: Give 1000 ml. D-5-W in 2 hrs. (When started at 9 a.m., the I.V. was regulated to flow at 125 gtts./min. Upon checking the bottle at 9:30 a.m. one finds 450 ml. left in the bottle.)

AVAILABLE: Abbott administration set.

SOLUTION: 450 ml. ÷ 1 1/2 hr. = 300 ml./hr.
                   300 ml. ÷ 60 min. = 5 ml./min.
                   5 ml. × 15 gtts. = 75 gtts./min.

ANSWER: At 9:30 a.m. regulate the flow of the fluid at 75 drops per minute, or less if indicated.

PROBLEM 4.   ORDERED: Give 1000 ml. D-5-W c̄ 40 mEq. potassium chloride (KCl) I.V. today.

AVAILABLE: Cutter administration set.

SOLUTION:

40 mEq. ÷ 20 mEq. = 2 hrs.
(Considering the fact that to prevent hyper-kalemia no more than 20 to 25 mEq. KCl per hour should be given intravenously to adults, this solution with 40 mEq. should run at least 2 hrs. However, other factors should be con-sidered when regulating the rate of flow in order to prevent dehydration, cardiac or re-spiratory embarrassment, and so forth.)

1000 ml. ÷ 2 hrs. = 500 ml./hr.
500 ml. × 20 gtts. = 10,000 gtts./hr.
10,000 gtts. ÷ 60 min. = 166 2/3 or 167 gtts./min.

ANSWER: Regulate I.V. to flow at a maximum of 167 drops per minute initially.

PROBLEM 5.   ORDERED: 2000 cc. D-5-W I.V. to run 24 hrs.
(When started at 10 a.m. the I.V. was regu-lated to flow at 14 gtts./min. See Problem 2 above. Now it is 12 noon the same day and 400 ml. remain in the first 1000 ml. bottle.)

AVAILABLE: Travenol administration set.

400 ml. ÷ 10 hrs. = 40 ml./hr.
40 ml. × 10 gtts. = 400 gtts./hr.
400 gtts. ÷ 60 min. = 6 2/3 or 7 gtts./min.

ANSWER: Regulate the I.V. to flow at 7 drops per minute.
(The first 1000 ml. was to run 12 hrs.; 10 of those 12 hrs. remain. Calculating on the basis of the 2000 ml. in 24 hrs. would result in greater fluid infusion in the first 12 hrs. than during the second 12 hrs.)

PROBLEM 6.   ORDERED: (Infant weighing 11 lbs.) 200 ml. Ringer's lac-tate I.V. q.d.

AVAILABLE: Microdrip (60 gtts./ml.) administration set.

200 ml. ÷ 24 hrs. = 8 1/3 ml./hr.
          8 1/3 ml. × 60 gtts. = 500 gtts./ml.
          500 gtts. ÷ 60 min. = 8 1/3 gtts./min.

(Note that when using 60 gtts./ml. microdrip sets, the desired ml./hr. equals the desired gtts./min because of dividing the *ml./hr.* by *60 min./hr.* then multiplying the *ml./hr.* by *60 gtts./ml.*)

ANSWER: Regulate the I.V. to flow at 8 drops per min.

Calculated infusion flow rates are guidelines only. Maintaining the calculated rate of flow does not relieve nurses of their responsibility to observe for indications of too rapid or too slow infusion. Fulfilling one's obligation to speed up, slow down, or stop an intravenous infusion at any time requires considerable nursing judgment based upon many factors which are far beyond the scope of this book.

Sometimes I.V. medications are added to a separate small volume I.V. fluid container and given by a method commonly called add-a-line or piggyback (P.B.). The needle on these add-a-line units usually is inserted into a rubber stoppered Y connector on the tubing of the main line. In order for the fluid containing the medication to flow, this container must be elevated above the level of the main line I.V. fluid container. Because these piggyback I.V. fluid containers contain 50, 100, or 250 ml. of fluid, this method is usually used for adults or older children only. Frequently the pharmacy adds the drug to the P.B. bag and properly labels them before they are sent to the nursing unit. However, on all units in most small hospitals and on some units in many large hospitals, nurses still prepare all I.V. medication solutions.

Sometimes two I.V.s may be infusing at the same time, using what is called a secondary set (Fig. 14). One or both may contain a medication. No problems of this kind are included because each I.V. is prepared and regulated as a separate I.V., using the control clamps above the point of the connection of the tubing.

PROBLEM 7. ORDERED: K.V.O. (keep vein open) with D-5-W. Pipracil 3 Gm. I.V. P.B. q.4h.

            AVAILABLE: Pipracil (piperacillin sodium) in 2, 3, and 4 Gm. vials. Travenol primary and P.B. administration sets and 50, 100, and 250 ml. P.B. solutions.

            DIRECTIONS: For I.M. use reconstitute q. Gm. with at least 2 ml. of diluent and there will be 1 Gm. in 2.5 ml. For I.V. use at least 5 ml./Gm. and give

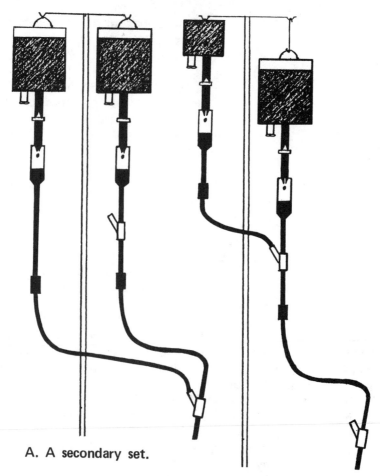

A. A secondary set.

B. A piggy back set.

FIGURE 14. Two I.V. infusion methods.

over 3–5 minutes or dilute further with at least 50 ml. and give over 30 minutes.

SOLUTION:

Add a minimum of 6 ml. diluent to a 3 Gm. vial in order to dissolve the drug. Use a 10 or 12 ml. syringe. There will be 7.5 ml. of reconstituted solution.

$$1 \text{ Gm.:2.5 ml.} = 3 \text{ Gm.:} x \text{ ml.}$$
$$1 x = 7.5 \text{ ml.}$$

A larger amount of diluent, up to the capacity of the vial, could be used. Add whatever amount of reconstituted drug is prepared to a 50 ml. P.B. bag of an appropriate solution.

Adding 7.5 ml. would result in a total of 57.5 ml. which should run 30 minutes.

$$57.5 \text{ ml.} \times 10 \text{ gtts.} = 575 \text{ gtts. in } 30 \text{ min.}$$
$$575 \text{ gtts.} \div 30 = 19 \text{ gtts./min.}$$

ANSWER: Add 6 ml. diluent to 3 Gm. vial of drug, add the 7.5 ml. reconstituted drug to a 50 ml. P.B. bag of solution, connect it to the primary set, and regulate at 19 drops per minute.

Often I.V. medications are given via heparin locks, either by I.V. push or in I.V. fluids given intermittently (Fig. 15). The procedure used in most health care agencies calls for the use of 2 to 5 ml. of sterile isotonic saline to clear the heparin from the needle and intracath before administering the I.V. medication and the use of the same amount after giving the medication. Flushing the lock with sterile isotonic saline before and after giving the medication is especially important when the medication is incompatible with heparin.

Filling the needle and intracath with an ordered or indicated amount of heparin solution is the final step. The amount of heparin solution needed varies with the type of heparin lock used. One kind needs 0.25 ml., another requires 0.6 ml. Special 1 ml. heparin flush Tubex ampules containing 10 or 100 units of heparin per ml. usually are available for this purpose. If not, it may be necessary to dilute the available heparin to a weaker strength.

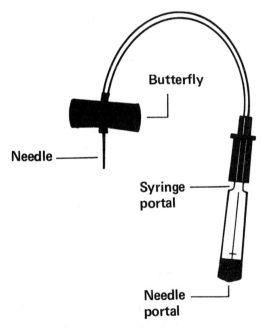

Butterfly

Needle ———

Syringe portal

Needle portal

FIGURE 15. Heparin lock.

PROBLEM 8.   ORDERED: (4-year-old child) Nafcillin 500 mg. intermittent I.V. q.4h. by heparin lock in 30 minutes.
Use 33 1/3 U./ml. heparin for lock.

AVAILABLE: Unipen (nafcillin sodium) 500 mg., 1 Gm., 1.5
Gm., 2 Gm., and 4 Gm. vials. Heparin 1 ml.
ampules with 1000 U.; I.V. P.B. fluid bags of
50, 100, and 250 ml. each; and Cutter primary
I.V. sets.

DIRECTIONS:

Vial size	Amount of diluent	Nafcillin solution
500 mg.	1.7 ml.	2 ml.
1 Gm.	3.4 ml.	4 ml.
2 Gm.	6.8 ml.	8 ml.

For direct injection dilute drug in 15 to 30 ml.
solution and inject over 5 to 10 minutes. For
intermittent I.V. add minimum of 49 ml. of
diluent to all sizes of vials except 4 Gm. to
which 97 ml. should be added. Administer
over at least 30 to 60 minutes to prevent vein
irritation. The drug is most stable at concentrations of 2 to 40 mg./ml.

SOLUTION: 2 mg.:1 ml. = 500 mg.:x ml.
$$2x = 500$$
$$x = 250 \text{ ml. maximum amount}$$
of drug solution

40 mg.:1 ml. = 500 mg.:x ml.
$$40x = 500$$
$$x = 12.5 \text{ ml. minimum amount}$$
of drug solution

52 ml. × 20 gtts./ml. = 1040 gtts. in 30 min.
1040 gtts. ÷ 30 min. = 34.67 gtts./min.

33 1/3 U.:1 ml. = 1000 U.:x ml.
$$33 \text{ 1/3 } x = 1000$$
$$x = 30 \text{ ml.}$$

ANSWER: Add 1.7 ml. diluent to 500 mg. vial of nafcillin.
Add 2 ml. of reconstituted nafcillin to 50 ml.
I.V. P.B. solution. Connect I.V. tubing to P.B.
bag, flush heparin lock with 2 ml. sterile isotonic saline or water, and connect I.V. tubing

76

to heparin lock. Adjust flow at 33 gtts./min. (Because the 2 ml. of drug added is less than 10% of the 50 ml., using 50 ml. as the total amount of drug solution would be accurate enough.)

Add 1 ml. of 1000 U./ml. heparin to a 30 ml. vial of sterile isotonic saline or water. Label "33 1/3 U./ml." for future use. After drug solution has infused, flush heparin lock with 2 ml. sterile isotonic saline or water, then add enough of the 33 1/3 U./ml. heparin to fill the lock being used.

There are many machines available that automatically regulate the flow of I.V. solutions at the rate to which they are set. These machines are almost always used for infants and small children and sometimes for older children and adults. With them it is possible to maintain very slow rates of flow. However, very close observation of pediatric patients and some adults for indications of too rapid infusion is imperative.

I.V. flow regulation machines can be classified into three general types: automatic controllers, volume delivery pumps, and syringe infusors. The automatic controllers, such as IVAC 230 and IVAC 260, regulate flow rate by drops per minute according to the drop size of the administration set being used. These machines do not exert pressure on the fluid being infused, and the actual flow rate may vary at times from the rate at which the machines are set. The flow rate can be affected by the position of the patient, the I.V. fluid bag, and/or the I.V. tubing, and by the size of the venipuncture needle or catheter.

Usually a fluid volume control chamber, for example, a Buretrol, a Soluset, or a Volutrol, are used with these machines. These chambers hold 100 or 150 ml. and have a calibrated mark for each 2 ml. Most often these chambers have microdrip (60 gtts./ml.) inlets. If a microdrip set is used, a machine set to deliver 20 gtts./min. should deliver 20 ml./hr.

In most instances the clamp above the chamber is opened and an hour's supply of fluid is added to the 5 or 10 ml. to be left in the chamber at the end of each hour in order to prevent air from getting into the tubing below. Limiting the amount of fluid that can be infused to an hour's supply is an added precaution against fluid overload.

Medications may be put into the rubber stoppered inlet ("Burette Port" in Fig. 16) on the fluid volume chambers with a syringe and needle or with a secondary I.V. P.B. set (see Fig. 16). Then the indicated amount of I.V. fluid is added from the primary fluid bottle or bag or from the P.B. bag. Medications can also be injected into any of the portals on the I.V. tubing below the pump. This is discussed below.

A general rule, especially for infants and children and adults on restricted fluids, is to infuse drugs at the same rate as the continuous I.V. fluid. The hourly ml. intake should not be increased appreciably.

Although 5 or 10 ml. should be left in volume control chambers at the end of each hour when giving the primary I.V. fluid, after a medication has been added to the chamber it should be emptied completely before adding another hour's supply (plus 5 or 10 ml.) to the chamber. This requires close observation so that air does not get into the tubing as the chamber is emptying.

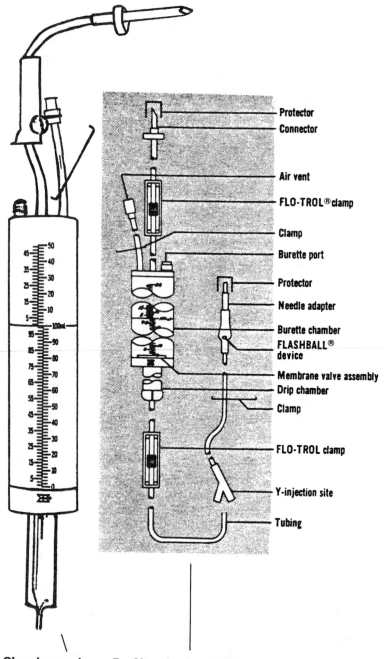

Protector
Connector
Air vent
FLO-TROL® clamp
Clamp
Burette port
Protector
Needle adapter
Burette chamber
FLASHBALL® device
Membrane valve assembly
Drip chamber
Clamp
FLO-TROL clamp
Y-injection site
Tubing

A. Chamber only.   B. Chamber and Tubing.

FIGURE 16. Fluid volume control chambers. (Courtesy of Travenol Laboratories, Inc.)

Whenever a drug is added to an I.V. system a label should be placed on the I.V. bag, the volume control chamber, or the infuser pump syringe containing the medication. Write the name and amount of drug and the time it was added. Remove the label when the drug has infused completely.

PROBLEM 9. ORDERED: (2 1/2-year-old child) Gentamicin 20 mg. I.V. q.8h. and D-5-0.2 N.S. at 35 ml./hr.

AVAILABLE: IVAC with microdrip Buretrol. Gentamicin 20 mg./2 ml. and 80 mg./2 ml. in Dosette syringes. P.B. bags of solution 50, 100, and 250 ml.

DIRECTIONS: Dilute in 50–200 ml. solution, less for children and infants, and give in 1/2 to 2 hours.

SOLUTION:

$$20 \text{ mg.}:2 \text{ ml.} = 20 \text{ mg.}:x \text{ ml}$$
$$20 x = 40$$
$$x = 2 \text{ ml. of } 20 \text{ mg.}/$$
$$2 \text{ ml. drug}$$

ANSWER: At the end of the hour there should be 10 ml. of the primary I.V. solution in the Buretrol, according to the hospital policy. The 2 ml. of drug could be added to the Buretrol and 23 ml. of the D-5-0.2 N.S. could be added to bring the total in the Buretrol to 35 ml. Continue the flow at 35 ml./hour. Let the Buretrol empty before adding 45 ml. (35 for the next hour and 10 reserve) of D-5-0.2 N.S.

The fluid volume delivery pumps, such as IVACs 600 and 630, Valley Lab, and IMED pumps, are the second general type of I.V. infusion machines. These *do* exert a pressure on the infusing fluid, therefore, the flow volume remains constant. They control the ml. per hour at the amount to which they are set. Some can be set to one-tenth of a ml. per hour. Either microdrip or macrodrip fluid volume chambers may be used with these machines. Medications may be introduced into any of the portals in the I.V. system.

PROBLEM 10. ORDERED: (1-year-old child) Amikin 50 mg. I.V. q.8h. and D-5-0.2 N.S.. at 30 ml./hr.

AVAILABLE: Amikin (amikacin sulfate) 100 mg./2 ml. vial. IMED with macrodrip Buretrol.

DIRECTIONS: For children use enough diluent to give over 30–60 minutes. For infants use enough diluent to give over 1–2 hours.

SOLUTION: The nurse decides to run the fluid with the drug for 1 hour.

ANSWER: Add 1 ml. of the drug to the end of hour 10 ml. residual in the Buretrol. Add 19 ml. of the primary I.V. solution to the Buretrol and continue flow at 30 ml./hour.

Syringe pumps are a third general type of machine for giving fluids intravenously. The Auto Syringe and Harvard infusor pumps are among the many available. These machines move the plunger of the syringe very slowly and at the rate set. The Auto Syringe pump will accommodate syringes from tuberculin to 35 ml. sizes. All other syringe pumps accommodate a 50 ml. syringe only. Some IMED volume control pumps can be converted easily to a syringe pump.

Syringe pumps are used when medications are to be given slowly over an extended period of time, when the volume of the drug solution is fairly small, and when no other continuous I.V. fluids are being given. The drugs can be given through a heparin lock or into various portals on the primary, secondary, or extension tubing.

Nurses need to consider the concentration and the rate of flow of the drug for two major reasons. First, the drug needs to be given at a rate and at a concentration that will ensure the attainment of therapeutic blood serum levels. However, many drugs are irritating to the veins and further dilution of the drug often reduces this irritation. Drug literature provides concentration recommendations. Sometimes it is acceptable to give drugs at concentrations greater than those recommended in order to prevent fluid overload, but certain drugs should not be given at greater than recommended concentrations.

Several recent research studies involving the administration of I.V. drugs to infants and children have shown that therapeutic serum levels were not always being attained when drugs were added high in the system, for example, into fluid volume control chambers.

In general, researchers have concluded that as the rate of flow and/or the volume of I.V. fluid containing the drug decreases, the closer the portal of injection of the drug solution into the I.V. system should be to the venipuncture site, in order to increase the amount of drug that is infused. Their reasons are as follows:

(1) Drugs have been found to adhere to filters and tubing throughout the system;
(2) drugs with a specific gravity lower than that of the primary I.V. solution tend to rise and remain in the I.V. tubing, and drugs with a specific gravity higher than that of the primary solution tend to fall and remain in any low loop of tubing; and
(3) the more distal from the patient's vein the drug is added to the system, the more drug is discarded when the primary I.V. tubing is changed to fulfill infection control measures.

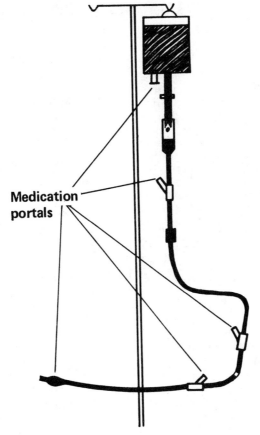

Medication portals

FIGURE 17 Possible medication injection sites.

For these reasons, the staff in some hospitals have protocols or policies to be used when selecting the drug injection site. See Figure. 17 for locations of injection sites not discussed above.

PROBLEM 11. ORDERED: (1-month-old, 11 lb. infant) Amikin 40 mg. I.V. q.12h. by syringe pump. D-5-0.2 N.S. to run at 15 ml./hr.

AVAILABLE: Amikin (amikacin sulfate) 100 mg./2 ml. vial; 50 ml., 100 ml., and 250 ml. I.V. P.B. bags of solution; IVAC; and Abbott primary and extension set.

DIRECTIONS: For infants use enough diluent to give over 1–2 hours.

SOLUTION:
$$100 \text{ mg.:2 ml.} = 40 \text{ mg.:}x \text{ ml.}$$
$$100 x = 80$$
$$x = 0.8 \text{ ml. drug}$$

The nurse decides to give the drug over a 2 hour period.

$$15 \text{ ml.}:1 \text{ hr.} = x \text{ ml.}:2 \text{ hrs.}$$
$$1 x = 30 \text{ ml.}$$

ANSWER: Put 0.8 ml. Amikin in 50 ml. syringe, fill to 30 ml., select appropriate injection site, and set syringe pump to run at 15 ml./hr.

PROBLEM 12. ORDERED: Aminophyline 50 mg./hour by continuous I.V. in D-5-W and with Harvard infusor.

AVAILABLE: Aminophylline 250 mg./10 ml. ampule and 500 mg./20 ml. ampule.

SOLUTION: Since this I.V. is to run continuously, the 500 mg./200 ml. ampule is used. The 20 ml. of drug is drawn into the 50 ml. Harvard infusor syringe. Then 30 ml. D-5-W is added to the syringe. The rate to which the infusor is to be set is calculated.

$$\begin{array}{cc} available & ordered \\ 500 \text{ mg.}:50 \text{ ml.} = & 50 \text{ mg.}:x \text{ ml.} \end{array}$$
$$500 x = 2500$$
$$x = 5 \text{ ml.}$$

ANSWER: Adjust the infusor to deliver 5 ml./hr.

The steps in I.V. medication problems are summarized below.

1. Amount of drug? (Doctor's order)
   A. May have to reconstitute drug.
   B. Usually have to convert gr., mg., Gm., U., or mEq. ordered to ml. to be given.
2. Put drug in how many ml. of I.V. fluid?
   A. This is affected by the type of administration (usually the nurse's decision):
   (1) Putting drug into total I.V. fluid sometimes.
   (2) Putting drug into P.B. bags is limited to the size of the bags unless some of the solution is withdrawn.
   (3) Putting drug into volume control chamber and adding primary fluid.
   (4) Giving drug by I.V. push into heparin lock or tubing portals is limited by the size of syringe, usually 20 ml. or 30 ml. maximum, minus the space to mix the drug and solution.
   (5) Giving drug by syringe pump is limited by size of the syringe, usually 50 ml.

B. This is affected by the concentration of the drug that is ordered or recommended and will be expressed as mg., Gm., U., or mEq. per ml.:
   (1) May be Doctor's order.
   (2) Literature may state recommended concentrations.
3. Rate of administration?
   A. May administer at rate nurse judges to be reasonable in gtts./min., ml./min., or ml./hr.:
      (1) Same rate as I.V. is running?
      (2) Different rate?
   B. Doctor may order or literature may recommend rate, e.g.,:
      (1) Amount of Gm. or mg./hours or minutes.
      (2) Give drug in 20 minutes or give drug in 1 hour.

CALCULATION OF FLUID NEEDS

Nurses need to be able to calculate fluid maintenance needs. One method that is used occasionally, especially with pediatric patients, is to use the guide of 1500 ml./m²/day. A 30 lb. child with a body surface area (B.S.A.) of 0.6 m² would need 900 ml./day or 37.5 ml./hr.

$$1500 \text{ ml.} \times 0.6 \text{m}^2 = 900 \text{ ml./day or } 37.5 \text{ ml./hr.}$$

Another guide many physicians consider to be more accurate and one which can be used for adults as well as children is as follows:

(1) 100 ml./kg. for first 10 kg.
(2) 50 ml./kg. for next 10 kg.
(3) 20 ml./kg. for weight over 20 kg.

A 220 lb. (100 kg.) man with no need for fluid restriction would need 1750 ml./day for maintenance or 73 ml./hr.

   100 kg.
 − 20 kg. (first and second 10 kg.)
   ─────
   80 kg.

$$20 \text{ ml.: } 1 \text{ kg.} = x \text{ ml.: } 80 \text{ kg.}$$
$$1x = 1600 \text{ ml.}$$

   1600 ml.
 + 150 ml. (100 ml. + 50 ml. for first and second 10 kg.)
   ─────────
   1750 ml./day or 73 ml./hr.

A 11 lb. (5 kg.) infant would need 500 ml./day or 21 ml./hr. or approximately 2 ounces q.3h. if on oral fluids.

$$100 \text{ ml.:} 1 \text{ kg.} = x \text{ ml.:} 5 \text{ kg.}$$
$$x = 500 \text{ ml./day or } 20.8 \text{ ml./hr.}$$

Using the first guide this 11 lb. (0.29 m²) infant would need 435 ml./day or 18 ml./hr.

$$1500 \text{ ml.} \times 0.29 \text{ m}^2 = 435 \text{ ml./day or } 18.125 \text{ ml./hr.}$$

Neonates (up to 1 month of age) require proportionately more fluid for their weight. Also, as one example, patients with cerebral edema may be given 2/3 or 3/4 of their maintenance needs.

CALCULATION OF CALORIES

An instance in which caloric intake may need to be calculated is when the patient is receiving I.V. fluids only. Usually the maximum amount of fluid given I.V. in a 24-hour period to an adult is 3,000 ml. Often this is a 5% dextrose solution. A 5% dextrose solution contains 5 Gm. of dextrose in every 100 ml. of solution. Using Formula B one can calculate the total calories that a patient will receive in 24 hours if he receives 3,000 ml. of D-5-W.

$$5 \text{ Gm.:100 ml.} = x \text{ Gm.:3,000 ml.}$$
$$100\,x = 15,000$$
$$x = 150 \text{ Gm.}$$
$$\underline{\times 4} \text{ (calories per Gm.)}$$
$$600 \text{ calories}$$

In a 24-hour period the patient would receive *only* 600 calories; these are carbohydrate calories only.

With hyperalimentation, when proteins (4 calories/Gm.) and fats (9 calories/Gm.) are given in addition to carbohydrates, it is possible to meet nutritional needs more adequately.

Practice Problems:

1. ORDERED: 1000 cc. D-5-W I.V. to run at 250 ml. per hr.

   AVAILABLE: Abbott administration set.

   ANSWER: _____

2. ORDERED: 1000 ml. D-5-W and 1000 ml. isotonic saline I.V. today.

   AVAILABLE: Cutter administration set. (Considering all the factors indicated one decides that this solution should run at least 6 hrs.)

   ANSWER: _____

3. ORDERED: 500 ml. D-5-W c̄ 40 mEq potassium chloride I.V. today.

   AVAILABLE: Travenol administration set.

   ANSWER: _____

4. ORDERED: 1000 ml. isotonic saline and 2000 ml. D-5-W I.V. to run 24 hrs.

   AVAILABLE: Abbott administration set. (I.V. was started at 10 a.m.)

   ANSWER: _____

5. ORDERED: Same as in Problem 4 above.

   AVAILABLE: Same as in Problem 4 above. (At noon the same day 700 ml. remain in the first bottle.)

   ANSWER: _____

6. ORDERED: (25 lb. infant) Add 400 ml. 1/6 M Ringer's lactate to I.V. and run 24 hrs.

   AVAILABLE: Microdrip (60 gtts./ml.) administration set.

   ANSWER: _____

7. ORDERED: 1000 ml. D-10-W I.V. to run from 9 a.m. to 3 p.m. today.

   AVAILABLE: Travenol administration set.

   ANSWER: _____

8. **ORDERED:** Same as in Problem 7 above.

   AVAILABLE: Same as in Problem 7 above. (At 10 a.m. there are 800 ml. in the bottle.)

   ANSWER: _____

9. **ORDERED:** Aminophylline 30 mg./hr. continuous I.V. with 500 mg./ 500 ml. D-5-W.

   AVAILABLE: Aminophylline 250 mg./10 ml. ampule and 500 mg./20 ml. ampule, IVAC volume control pump, and 500 ml. bags of D-5-W.

   ANSWER: _____

10. **ORDERED:** (2-year-old child) Aminophylline 8 mg./hr. continuous I.V. in D-5-W. (Dilute at 1 mg./ml.)

    AVAILABLE: Aminophylline 250 mg./10 ml. ampules, IMED volume control pump, and 50, 100, and 250 ml. I.V. P.B. bags of D-5-W.

    ANSWER: _____

11. **ORDERED:** Regular Insulin 1.0 U./hr. by continuous I.V. by heparin lock for 24-hour administration.

    AVAILABLE: Regular Insulin 100 U./ml. and Harvard infusor.

    ANSWER: _____

12. **ORDERED:**   (14-year-old child) Valium 5 mg. I.V. q.3–4h. p.r.n. and D-5-0.45-NaCl continuous I.V. at 30 ml./hr.

   AVAILABLE: Valium (diazepam) 5 mg./ml. in 2 ml. syringes, 2 ml. ampules, and 10 ml. vials; Travenol primary I.V. sets; and 250, 500, and 1000 ml. bottles of D-5-0.45-NaCl.

   DIRECTIONS: Inject slowly I.V., no faster than 5 mg./min., and if can't inject directly put into I.V. tubing, as near needle as possible.

   ANSWER: _____

13. **ORDERED:**   Neo-Synephrine 0.5 mcg./min. continuous I.V. in D-5-W.

   AVAILABLE: Neo-Synephrine HCl 1% (10 mg./ml.) ampules and IMED volume control pump. Nurse decides to put 5 mg. in 500 ml. D-5-W.

   ANSWER: _____

14. **ORDERED:**   (3-year-old child) Gentamycin 15 mg. I.V. q.8h. and Ringer's Lactate at 15 ml./hr.

   AVAILABLE: Gentamycin sulfate Dossette syringes 20 mg./2 ml., IMED controller with microdrip Soluset. Hospital policy calls for 10 ml. I.V. fluid reserve in Soluset at the end of each hour.

   DIRECTIONS: Dilute in 50–200 ml., less for children and infants, and give in 1/2–2 hours.

   ANSWER: _____

15. ORDERED: Heparin 500 U./hr. by continuous I.V.

    AVAILABLE: Heparin 1 ml. Tubex syringes with 1000, 2500, 5000,
                  7500, 10,000, 15,000, and 20,000 U./ml. and Harvard
                  infusor.

    ANSWER: _____

16. ORDERED: (Newborn) Vira-A 60 mg. I.V. over 24-hour period q.d. for
                  10 days.

    AVAILABLE: Vira-A 5 ml.-1 Gm. vial (200 mg./ml.). IMED volume con-
                  trol pump with 0.1 ml. settings and with 150 ml. macro-
                  drip Buretrol.

    DIRECTIONS: Need minimum of 2.22 ml. I.V. solution/mg. of drug for
                  complete solubilization. Warm to 35–40°C or 95–100°F.

    ANSWER: _____

17. ORDERED: Dobutamine 250 mcg./minute continuous I.V.

    AVAILABLE: Dobutrex (dobutamine HCl) 250 mg. vials and Harvard
                  infusor.

    DIRECTIONS: Add 10 ml. diluent and if not dissolved add another 10
                  ml. diluent. May dilute up to 50 ml.

    ANSWER: _____

18. ORDERED: Unipen 500 mg. I.V. q.4h. and continuous D-5-0.45-NaCl
                  at 40 ml./hr.

    AVAILABLE: Unipen (nafcillin sodium) 500 mg. vials; 50, 100, and
                  250 ml. P.B. bags of solution; and Abbott primary and
                  secondary I.V. tubing sets.

    DIRECTIONS: Dilute to maximum concentration of 40 mg./ml. or less
                  and give over at least 30–60 minutes.

    ANSWER: _____

19. ORDERED: (12-year-old child) Chloromycetin 500 mg. I.V. push
                  q.6h. via heparin lock.

    AVAILABLE: Chloromycetin (chloramphenicol sodium succinate)
                  1 Gm. vials for I.V. use only.

    DIRECTIONS: Give 10% (100 mg./ml.) solution over 1 minute or add
                  10 ml. diluent. When reconstituted as directed there
                  will be 100 mg./ml. or 1 Gm. in 10 ml.

    ANSWER: _____

20. ORDERED: Amicar 1 Gm./hr. into continuous I.V. of D-5-W at
                  K.V.O. otherwise.

    AVAILABLE: Amicar (aminocaproic acid) 20 ml. vial with 250 mg./ml.
                  and Harvard infusor. Hospital practice calls for infu-
                  sion into Y portal nearest venipuncture.

    ANSWER: _____

21. ORDERED: Cefadyl 1 Gm. I.V. q.6h. by intermittent I.V. via heparin lock in 20 minutes.

    AVAILABLE: Cefadyl (cephapirin sodium) 500 mg., 1 Gm., and 2 Gm. vials; 50 ml. P.B. I.V. solution; and Travenol primary I.V. administration set.

    DIRECTIONS: Reconstitute 500 mg. and 1 Gm. vials with 1 ml. or 2 ml. diluent to get 500 mg./1.2 ml. For I.V. use dilute 500 mg., 1 Gm., or 2 Gm. with 10 ml. or more diluent and give over 3 to 5 minutes or by intermittent I.V. infusion.

    ANSWER: _____

22. ORDERED: (6-year-old child) Cleocin 200 mg. I.V. q.8h. and D-5-0.45-NaCl continuous I.V. running at 50 ml./hr.

    AVAILABLE: Cleocin (clindamycin phosphate) 150 mg./ml. in 2 and 4 ml. ampules. IVAC controller with 150 ml. microdrip Buretrol and extension tubing. All sizes of P.B. fluids. Hospital policy dictates injection into the last portal on the primary I.V. tubing for fluids running at this rate.

    DIRECTIONS: Dilute to 300 mg. in 50 ml. or more fluid.

Dose	Diluent	Time
300 mg.	50 ml.	10 min.
600 mg.	100 ml.	20 min.
900 mg.	150 ml.	30 min.
1200 mg.	200 ml.	45 min.

    ANSWER: _____

23. ORDERED: (5-year-old child) Ticar 1 Gm. I.V. q.4h. via heparin lock and intermittent drip.

    AVAILABLE: Ticar (ticarcillin disodium) 1, 3, and 6 Gm. vials; 50, 100, and 250 ml. P.B. bags of I.V. solution; and Abbott primary I.V. set.

    DIRECTIONS: Dilute to 1 Gm./20 ml. or more to reduce vein irritation. Most stable at concentrations of 10 mg./ml. to 50 mg./ml. Give by intermittent drip over 30 min. to 2 hours. The nurse decides to give in 1 hour.

    ANSWER: _____

24. ORDERED: (2-year-old child) Septra 50 mg. I.V. q.8h. and I.V. of D-5-W at K.V.O. with IVAC controller and microdrip Soluset.

    AVAILABLE: Septra (trimethoprim and sulfamethoxazole). Each 5 ml. ampule contains 80 mg. t (16 mg./ml.) and 400 mg. s (80 mg./ml.). (Amount ordered is based on t component of the drug.)

    DIRECTIONS: Mix with D-5-W only. No rapid or bolus injection. Each 5 ml. ampule should be added to 125 ml. D-5-W or as little as 75 ml. if on restricted fluids. Give over 60–90 minutes. The nurse decides to give in 60 minutes.

    ANSWER: _____

CHAPTER 4

CHILDREN'S DOSAGES

Only physicians may prescribe dosages of medications, but nurses must know if ordered dosages are within the safe range for the individual patient before they carry out the order. This is especially true for infants and children. Since some textbooks do not include dosages for infants and children, nurses may need to determine these from the known, usual adult dosages.

In past years, Young's, Fried's, and Clark's rules were commonly used for determining dosages for infants and children. These rules, rarely used today, are included for the convenience of some instructors, but problems involving their use have been omitted. When used, the rules should serve as rough guides to determining approximate child dosages. It should be noted that Young's or Fried's rules do not allow for such important factors as the child's weight or size.

YOUNG'S RULE (for children from 1 or 2 to 12 years)
$$\frac{\text{Age in years}}{\text{Age plus 12}} \times \text{Adult dose} = \text{Child's dose}$$

FRIED'S RULE (for infants and children up to 1 or 2 years)
$$\frac{\text{Age in months}}{150} \times \text{Adult dose} = \text{Infant's or child's dose}$$

CLARK'S RULE (for infants or children)
$$\frac{\text{Weight in pounds}}{150} \times \text{Adult dose} = \text{Infant's or child's dose}$$

In addition to weight or size, the physiologic and pathologic conditions must also be considered, as must the nature of the drug. For instance, children have relatively less tolerance for narcotics than adults do. Also, administering the correct dosage to infants under two months is most critical because their kidneys and liver are immature. This remains a factor until age two.

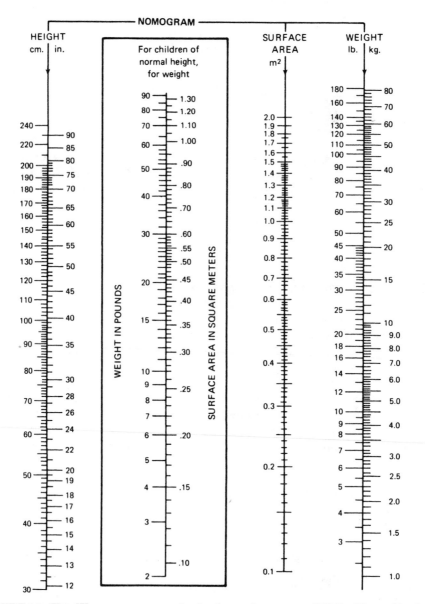

FIGURE 18. The West nomogram for body surface area (BSA). (From Shirkey, H. C., *Drug therapy*. In Vaughn, V. C., III, and McKay, R. J., eds., *Nelson's Textbook of Pediatrics*, ed. 11, W. B. Saunders Co., Philadelphia, 1979, p. 2055.)

Some physicians believe that use of body surface area (BSA) is the most accurate method of estimating safe dosages for infants and children weighing less than 10 kilograms because BSA is thought to be more closely related to infants' or children's metabolism than is their weight. However, the use of BSA for calculating dosage for infants weighing less than 10 kilograms will result in excessive dosages. The most commonly used BSA rule is:

$$\frac{\text{Surface area in square meters} \times \text{Adult dose}}{1.7} = \text{Infant's or child's dose}$$

To determine BSA in square meters (m²) one uses a nomogram (Fig. 18). To use a nomogram (1) plot the child's height and weight on the left and right vertical columns; (2) place a straight-edge on the vertical height and weight lines where these lines intersect the plotted height and weight shown by short horizontal lines; and (3) determine the BSA in m² at the point at which the straight edge crosses the surface area (SA) scale. If a child's weight is 24 pounds and his height is 28 inches, his BSA is 0.48 m². If the child is of normal height for weight, weight alone can be used to determine BSA using the boxed area on the nomogram.

Pharmaceutical companies rarely state recommended dosages for children, but sometimes state a specific amount of drug per m² of BSA. Sometimes they state proper dosages per m² and per kilogram of weight. Most often they state only recommended dosages as the amount of drug per kg. of body weight per day in divided doses.

Remember that 1 kilogram equals 2.2 pounds. Therefore, an adult weighing 220 pounds weighs 100 kilograms.

$$1 \text{ kg.}:2.2 \text{ lbs.} = x \text{ kg.}:220 \text{ lbs.}$$
$$2.2 \, x = 220$$
$$x = 100 \text{ kg.}$$

An infant weighing 11 pounds weighs 5 kilograms.

$$\frac{1 \text{ kg.}}{2.2 \text{ lbs.}} = \frac{x \text{ kg.}}{11 \text{ lbs.}}$$
$$2.2 \, x = 11$$
$$x = 5 \text{ kg.}$$

Examples:

PROBLEM 1.   ORDERED: (6-year-old child, weight 42 lbs., height 45 in.) Morphine sulfate 4 mg. I.M. q.4h. p.r.n. for pain.

ADULT DOSE: Usual is 15 mg.; range is 8–20 mg.

SOLUTION: *SURFACE AREA RULE* (The nomogram was used to determine that this child's BSA is 0.78 m²)

$$\frac{0.78 \text{ m}^2 \times 15 \text{ mg.}}{1.7} = x$$
$$x = \frac{11.70}{1.7}$$
$$x = 6.88 \text{ mg.}$$

The ordered dose is reasonable since it is considerably less than the 7.06 mg. determined to be within safe limits—but remember that this is a narcotic.

PROBLEM 2:   ORDERED: (15-month-old baby, weight 28 1/2 lbs., normal height for weight)
Demerol (meperdine) 5 mg. I.M. q.4h. p.r.n.

ADULT DOSE: 50–100 mg. q.4h.

SOLUTION: *SURFACE AREA RULE* (The nomogram scale for children of normal height for weight was used to determine the baby's BSA to be 0.58 m²)

$$\frac{0.58 \, m^2 \times 100 \, mg.}{1.7} = x$$

$$x = \frac{58}{1.7}$$

$$x = 34.12 \, mg.$$

The amount ordered is within safe limits. *Note*: this also is a narcotic.

PROBLEM 3.   ORDERED: (2-month-old infant, height 22 in., weight 3.5 kg.)
Cleocin 75 mg. I.M. q.6h.

AVAILABLE: Clindamycin phosphate (Cleocin) 150 mg./ml. in 2 and 4 ml. ampules.

DIRECTIONS: Children over 1 month give 15–25 mg./kg./day in 3 or 4 equal doses up to a maximum of 25–40 mg./kg./day, or, give 350 mg./m²/day up to a maximum of 450 mg./m²/day. Give minimum of 300 mg./day regardless of weight.

The amount ordered is reasonable. Use of the maximum of 40 mg./kg./day does give an amount less than that ordered. Use of the maximum of 450 mg./m²/day gives an amount of 105.75 mg., less than the amount ordered. However, directions also say to give a minimum of 300 mg./day regardless of weight. The nomogram was used to determine that the infant's BSA is 0.235 m². Directions in this instance did not require the use of the Surface Area Rule with the adult dose, nor would it be possible to use this rule without stating the adult dose.

SOLUTION 1:   40 mg.:1 kg. = x mg.:3.5 kg.
                               1 x = 140 mg.

SOLUTION 2:   450 mg.:1 m² = x mg.:0.235 m²
                               1 x = 105.75 mg.

Therefore, give this infant 0.5 ml. Cleocin I.M. q. 6h.

$$150 \, mg.:1 \, ml. = 75 \, mg.:x \, ml.$$
$$150 \, x = 75$$
$$x = 0.5 \, ml.$$

PROBLEM 4. ORDERED: (1-week-old infant, weight 4000 Gm., length 18 in.)
Chloromycetin 25 mg. I.V. q.6h.

AVAILABLE: Chloramphenicol sodium succinate (Chloromycetin) 100 mg./ml. when reconstituted as directed.

DIRECTIONS: Newborn to 2 weeks give 25 mg./kg./day in divided doses every 6 hours. Children and adults give 50 mg./kg./day in 4 divided doses with maximum of 100 mg./kg./day.

SOLUTION:

$$25 \text{ mg.}:1 \text{ kg.} = x \text{ mg.}:4 \text{ kg.}$$
$$1x = 100 \text{ mg.}$$

The amount ordered is equal to the recommended dose of 25 mg./kg./day. Therefore, give this infant 0.25 ml. Chloromycetin in appropriate amount of I.V. solution q.6h.

Practice Problems:

1. ORDERED: (8-year-old child, weight 50 lbs., height 48 in.)
0.5 Gm. Gantrisin (sulfisoxazole and phenazopyridine HCl) p.o. q.4h.

AVAILABLE: 0.5 Gm. Gantrisin tablets.

ADULT DOSE: 1 Gm. q.4h.

ANSWER: _____

2. ORDERED: (1-year-old baby, weight 17.5 lbs., normal height for weight)
Aspirin 1 gr. p.o. q.4h.

AVAILABLE: Aspirin (acetylsalicylic acid) gr. 1 tablets.

ADULT DOSE: 5–10 gr. q.4h.

ANSWER: _____

3. ORDERED: (1-year-old child, weight 22 lbs.)
Mezlin 0.5 Gm. I.V. q.4h.

   AVAILABLE: Mezlin (mezlocillin sodium) 1 Gm. vial.

   DIRECTIONS: Infants 0–1 week give 75 mg./kg. q.12h.; infants 1 week–1 month give 75 mg./kg. q.8h.; children 1 month–12 years give 50 mg./kg. q.4h.

   ANSWER: _____

4. ORDERED: (5-year-old child, weight 43 lbs., height 41 in.)
Pipracil 2 Gm. I.V. q.6h.

   AVAILABLE: Pipracil (piperacillin sodium) 2 Gm. vial.

   ADULT DOSE: 3–4 Gm. q.4–6h. up to 24 Gm./day.

   ANSWER: _____

5. ORDERED: (10-year-old male, weight 64 lbs., height 3 ft. 19 in.)
Cortisone 12.5 mg. p.o. q.i.d. maintenance dose.

   AVAILABLE: Cortisone acetate 25 mg. scored tablets.

   ADULT DOSE: As much as 300 mg. first day, 200 mg. second day, and 100 mg. daily thereafter.

   ANSWER: _____

6. ORDERED: Same as problem 5.

   AVAILABLE: Same as problem 5.

   DIRECTIONS: Maintenance dose for children is 0.7 mg./kg./day divided into 3 doses.

   ANSWER: _____

7. ORDERED: (9-month-old infant, weight 8 kg., height 70 cm.)
Cleocin 75 mg. I.V. q.6h.

   AVAILABLE: Cleocin (clindamycin phosphate) 150 mg./ml. in 2 and 4 ml. ampoules.

   DIRECTIONS: Children over 1 month give 15–25 mg./kg./day in 3–4 doses up to maximum of 25–40 mg./kg./day, or, give 350 mg./m²/day up to maximum of 450 mg./m²/day. Give minimum of 300 mg./day regardless of weight.

   ANSWER: _____

8. ORDERED: (4-year-old child, weight 20 kg., normal height for weight)
Digoxin 0.05 mg. I.V. b.i.d.

   AVAILABLE: Lanoxin (digoxin) 0.5 mg./2 ml. and 0.1 mg./1 ml.

   ADULT DOSE: Average divided I.V. digitalizing dose is 1.0 mg. (0.5–1.5 mg.)/day; maintenance dose is 0.5 mg. (0.25–0.75 mg.)/day.

   ANSWER: _____

9. ORDERED: (7-year-old child, weight 40 lbs., height 100 cm., with mild renal failure)
Mandol 500 mg. I.V. q.6h.

   AVAILABLE: Mandol (cefamandole nafate) 500 mg. vial.

   DIRECTIONS: Give children and infants 50–100 mg./kg./day divided q.4–8h. With mild renal impairment give 0.75–1.5 Gm. q.6h.

   ANSWER: _____

10. ORDERED: (2-year-old child, weight 8.8 kg., with cellulitis)
                  Cefamandole 300 mg. I.V. q.6h.

    AVAILABLE: Cefamandole nafate 500 mg. vial.

    DIRECTIONS: For cellulitis give children 100–150 mg./kg./day.

    ANSWER: _____

11. ORDERED: (5 1/2-month-old infant, weight 4.4 kg., has meningitis)
                  Ampicillin 125 mg. I.V. q.4h.
                  Chloramphenicol 100 mg. I.V. q.6h.

    AVAILABLE: Omnipen-N (ampicillin sodium) 125 mg. vial.
                  Chloromycetin (chloramphenicol sodium succinate)
                  100 mg./ml. when reconstituted as directed.

    DIRECTIONS: For children with meningitis give 200 mg./kg./day of
                  ampicillin in divided doses and give 100 mg./kg./day of
                  chloramphenicol in divided doses.

    ANSWER: _____

12. ORDERED: (9-year-old child, weight 75 lbs.)
                  Cefadyl 500 mg. I.V. q.6h.

    AVAILABLE: Cefadyl (cephapirin sodium) 500 mg. vial.
                  Reconstitute 500 mg. vial with 1 ml. diluent to get 500
                  mg./1.2 ml.

    DIRECTIONS: Give children 40–80 mg./kg./day depending on age,
                  weight, and severity of infection.

    ANSWER: _____

CHAPTER 5

REVIEW PROBLEMS

$$\frac{1 \; gm}{1000 \; mg} = \frac{.6}{}$$

1. 0.6 Gm. = ? gr.

$$\frac{.6 \; gm}{x \; gr} = = \frac{1 \; gm}{15}$$

3.6

$\frac{.6}{9.6}$

$9 =$

$9 \; gr$ 10

ANSWER: _____

2. 50 mg. = ? Gm.

ANSWER: _____ .05 _____

3. 1 1/2 gr. = ? mg.

$gr = 60 \; mg$

$1.5 \; gr$

$90 \; mg$

ANSWER: _____

4. 100 mg. = ? gr.

$1000 \; mg = 15$

ANSWER: _____ 1.5 gr _____

5. ORDERED: Quinidine 3 gr. I.M. stat.   3 gr   1

   AVAILABLE: 10 cc. vial of quinidine gluconate injection 80 mg. per ml.

   ANSWER: _____

6. ORDERED: 2000 ml. D-5-W I.V. in 24 hrs.

   AVAILABLE: Abbott administration set.

   ANSWER: _____

7. ORDERED: Lente insulin 50 units 1 hr. a.c. breakfast tomorrow.

   AVAILABLE: Insulin zinc suspension (lente) 100 U. and 100 U. scale insulin syringe and hypodermic syringes.

   ANSWER   _____

8. ORDERED: ASA 0.6 Gm. q.3-to-4h. p.r.n. for pain or fever over 102°F.

   AVAILABLE: Acetylsalicylic acid (ASA) 5 gr. tablets.

   ANSWER: _____

9. ORDERED: Adrenalin 0.4 mg. "H" q.3h. p.r.n. for asthma.

   AVAILABLE: 30 ml. vial epinephrine (Adrenalin) 1:2000.

   ANSWER: _____

10. **ORDERED:** 25% alcohol cooling sponge p.r.n. (Assume 1 qt. is needed each time.)

   AVAILABLE: 70% isopropyl alcohol.

   ANSWER: _____

11. **ORDERED:** Nembutal 100 mg., atropine 0.4 mg., and Demerol 75 mg. "H" on call to surgery.

   AVAILABLE: 2 ml. ampules of sodium pentobarbital (Nembutal) 1 1/2 gr. in 2 ml., multiple-dose vials of atropine gr. 1/150 per ml., and 2 ml. ampules of meperidine hydrochloride (Demerol) 50 mg. per ml.

   ANSWER: _____

12. **ORDERED:** (Infant) Kantrex 150 mg. I.M.q. 12 h.

   AVAILABLE: Kanamycin sulfate (Kantrex) solution 0.5 Gm. per 2 ml.

   ANSWER: _____

13. **ORDERED:** Kaon Elixir 15 mEq. t.i.d.

   AVAILABLE: A 4 oz. bottle of potassium gluconate (Kaon) 40 mEq. per oz.

   ANSWER: _____

14. ORDERED: Isotonic sodium chloride (NaCl) enema stat and p.r.n. (Prepare 2 qts.)

     AVAILABLE: Sodium chloride crystals.

     ANSWER: _____

15. ORDERED: Aqueous buffered penicillin G 400,000 U. I.M. q.4h.

     AVAILABLE: A 20 ml. vial of buffered penicillin G potassium 1,000,000 U. To get 250,000 U. per ml. add 3.6 ml. diluent.

     ANSWER: _____

16. ORDERED: Ferrous sulfate 300 mg. p.o. t.i.d.

     AVAILABLE: Ferrous sulfate gr. ii ss tablets

     ANSWER: _____

17. ORDERED: Elixir of phenobarbital 30 mg. p.o. stat.

     AVAILABLE: Elixir of phenobarbital gr. ī per dram

     ANSWER: _____

18. ORDERED: Atropine sulfate gr. 1/200 I.M. stat.

     AVAILABLE: Atropine sulfate gr. 1/150/ml. multidose vial

     ANSWER: _____

19. **ORDERED:** Regular insulin 15 U and N.P.H. insulin 30 U. 1/2 hr. a.c. breakfast every a.m.

   AVAILABLE: Regular insulin 100 U and N.P.H. insulin 100 U. No insulin syringes available.

   ANSWER: _____

20. **ORDERED:** Phenobarbital 1/2 gr. p.o. q.i.d.

   AVAILABLE: Phenobarbital sodium tablets 30 mg. and 60 mg.

   ANSWER: _____

21. **ORDERED:** (2 kg. premature infant) Solu-Medrol 2 mg. I.V. q.6h. and IVAC set at 2 ml./hr.

   AVAILABLE: Methylprednisolone sodium succinate (Solu-Medrol) in Mix-O-Vial that when reconstituted contains 40 mg. in 1 ml. and an Auto-Syringe.

   DIRECTIONS: Hospital policy for flow rates less than 10 ml./hr. is to use tubing portal nearest patient and a syringe pump.

   ANSWER: _____

22. **ORDERED:** (1-year-old infant) Phenobarbital 5 mg. p.o. stat.

   AVAILABLE: Phenobarbital sodium tablets 30 mg.

   ANSWER: _____

23. ORDERED: (1-year-old child) Ampicillin 100 mg. I.V. q.6h. D-5-0.2NS at 24 ml./hour.

    AVAILABLE: Ampicillin sodium 125 mg. vial. IVAC with Volutrol microdrip chamber and I.V. extension tubing.

    DIRECTIONS: Add 1 ml. to 125 mg. vial to get 125 mg./ml. For direct I.V. add 5 ml. diluent to 125 mg. vial and give over 3–5 minutes. Hospital policy for 20–30 ml./hr. flow rate is to give by syringe into last portal on primary tubing at 1 ml./minute and to use syringe pumps for more than 5 ml. drug solution.

    ANSWER: _____

24. ORDERED: (1-year-old child, weight 24 lbs., height 30 in.)

    Ceclor 75 mg. p.o. q.8h. (Is dose correct?)

    AVAILABLE: Ceclor (cefaclor) oral suspension 125 mg./5 ml. and 250 mg./5 ml.

    DIRECTIONS: Adult dose is 250 mg. q.8h. up to 4 Gm./day. Child dose is 20 mg./kg./day divided into q.8h. doses.

    ANSWER: _____

25. ORDERED: (5-year-old child, weight 45 lbs.)

    Vistaril 20 mg. I.M. stat. (Is dose correct?)

    AVAILABLE: Vistaril (hydroxyzine HCl) 25 mg./1 ml. vial.

    DIRECTIONS: Child dose is 0.5 mg./lb.

    ANSWER: _____

26. **ORDERED:**   K.V.O. with D-5-1/2 NS. Ampicillin 500 mg. I.V. q.6h. at 8-2-8-2 and Cleocin 400 mg. I.V. q.6h. at 12-6-12-6, each within 1 hour.

AVAILABLE: Drip chamber yielding 10 gtts./ml. Cleocin (clindamycin phosphate) 150 mg./ml. in 2 and 4 ml. ampules. (Clindamycin should be diluted to no more than 300 mg./50 ml.) Polycillin-N (ampicillin sodium) 500 mg. in vials and adding 1.8 ml. diluent yields 2 ml. reconstituted solution. (Polycillin-N is to be administered within 1 hour after reconstitution.) D-5-W in 50, 100, and 150 ml. piggyback containers.

ANSWER: _____

27. **ORDERED:**   (900 gm. premature infant) Heparin 50 units I.V. push q.6h. and I.V. at 1 ml./hour.

AVAILABLE: IMED volume delivery pump and heparin 100 units/ml. in Tubex syringe.

DIRECTIONS: May be given as available or may be diluted. Policy calls for use of flashball, the tubing portal nearest the patient.

ANSWER: _____

28. **ORDERED:**   1000 D-5-W I.V. to run 8 a.m.–4 p.m. today. (At 10 a.m. there is 600 ml. left in the bag.)

AVAILABLE: Cutter administration set.

ANSWER: _____

29. ORDERED: Lente insulin 35 U. and regular insulin 10 U. 20 min. a.c. every a.m.

    AVAILABLE: Lente insulin 100 U. and regular insulin 100 U. and no insulin syringe.

    ANSWER: _____

30. ORDERED: (1-year-old infant) Prostaphlin 125 mg. q.6h. I.V. at a maximum of 50 mg./hour and D-5-0.2NaCl to run at 24 ml./hour with IVAC and microdrip Soluset.

    AVAILABLE: Prostaphlin (oxacillin sodium) in 250 mg. vials. (The drug is to be given at a concentration of 0.5 to 2.0 mg./ml.)

    ANSWER: _____

31. ORDERED: Aspirin 0.6 Gm. prn headache.

    AVAILABLE: Aspirin gr. v tablets.

    ANSWER: _____

32. ORDERED: Morphine Sulfate 1/4 gr. "H" q 3–4 hrs. prn pain.

    AVAILABLE: Morphine Sulfate 1/8 gr./ml.

    ANSWER: _____

33. ORDERED: 500 ml. of a 2% Boric Acid solution.

    AVAILABLE: 600 ml. of 5% Boric Acid solution.

    ANSWER: _____

34. ORDERED: 2 liters of 20% Sodium Bicarconate solution.

    AVAILABLE: Sodium Bicarbonate powder.

    ANSWER: _____

APPENDIX **A**

SYSTEMS OF MEASUREMENT

HOUSEHOLD MEASURES

Nurses may use or teach the use of household articles for the measurement of drugs or solutions of drugs. Since household measures are not accurate, one should not substitute household equivalents for metric or apothecaries' measurements ordered by the physician. Note that all household measures are volume measurements. Occasionally, however, a volume measure must be used as a substitute for a weight measure. The equivalents below are approximate, not accurate.

TABLE 2. Approximate household equivalents

HOUSEHOLD	HOUSEHOLD	
15–16 drops (gtts.)	1/4 teaspoon (tsp.)	
2 teaspoons	1 dessertspoon (dssp.)	
3 teaspoons	1 tablespoon (tbsp.)	
2 tablespoons	1 fluid ounce (fl. oz.)	
3 dessertspoons	1 fluid ounce	
6 fluid ounces	1 teacup	
8 fluid ounces	1 glass of 1 measuring cup	

HOUSEHOLD	APOTHECARIES'	METRIC
1 drop	1 minim	0.06–0.07 ml.
1 teaspoon	1 fluid dram	4 or 5 ml.
1 tablespoon	4 fluid drams	15 or 16 ml.
2 tablespoons	1 fluid ounce	30 or 32 ml.
3 dessertspoons	1 fluid ounce	30 or 32 ml.
1 teacup	6 fluid ounces	180 or 192 ml.
1 glass or 1 measuring cup	8 fluid ounces or 1/2 pint	240 or 250 ml.
2 glasses or 2 measuring cups	16 fluid ounces or 1 pint	480 or 500 ml.
4 glasses or 4 measuring cups	1 quart	960 or 1000 ml.

APOTHECARIES' SYSTEM

The apothecaries' system is one of several different and confusing old English systems of weights and measurement. The basic unit of weight in the apothecaries' system is the grain, originally the weight of a grain of wheat. The basic unit of fluid measure in this system is the minim, the approximate amount of water that would weigh one grain. Other units of measure that may be used in drug administration are given in Table 3. Additional apothecaries' units of measure that are rarely or never used by nurses in the administration of drugs are not included.

TABLE 3. Apothecaries' equivalents

WEIGHT UNITS	
60 grains (gr.)	1 dram (з or dr.)
8 drams (з) or 480 grains	1 ounce (з)
12 ounces (з)	1 pound (lb.)
FLUID UNITS	
60 minims (m.)	1 fluid dram (fl.з)
8 fluid drams (fl.з) or 480 minims (m.)	1 fluid ounce (fl.з)
16 fluid ounces (fl.з)	1 pint (pt. or O.)
2 pints (pt. or O.)	1 quart (qt.)
4 quarts (qt.)	1 gallon (C or gal.)
WEIGHT UNITS*	**FLUID UNITS***
1 grain (gr.)	1 minim (m.)
60 grains (gr.)	1 fluid dram (fl.з), 60 m.
480 grains (gr.)	1 fluid ounce (fl.з), 480 m.

*The above apothecaries' weight-fluid units are approximate equivalents only but, when needed, these approximations are acceptable for the preparation and administration of solutions and drugs.

TABLE 4. Approximate apothecaries' metric volume equivalents

APOTHECARIES'	METRIC
1 minim (m.)	0.06–0.07 milliliter (ml.)
4 m.	0.25 ml.
8 m.	0.5 ml.
15 or 16 m.	1 ml. or 1 cubic centimeter (cc.)
1 fluid dram or 60 or 64 m.	4 ml.
1 fluid ounce (fl. oz.) or 8 fl. drams	30 or 32 ml.
1 pint (pt.) or 16 fl. oz.	480 or 500 ml.
1 quart (qt.) or 32 fl. oz.	960 or 1000 ml. or 1 liter (L.)
1 gallon (gal.) or 128 fl. oz.	3840 or 4000 ml. or 4 L.

TABLE 5. Commonly used approximate apothecaries' metric weight equivalents

APOTHECARIES'	METRIC
1/60, 1/64, or 1/65 grain (gr.)	1 milligram (mg.) or 1000 micrograms (mcg.)
1 gr.	0.06, 0.064, or 0.065 gram (Gm.)
1 gr.	60, 64, or 65 mg.
1 gr.	60,000, 64,000, or 65,000 mcg.
5 gr.	0.3 or 0.33 Gm.
10 gr.	0.6 or 0.67 Gm.
15 or 16 gr.	1 Gm.
1 dram	4 Gm.
1 ounce	30 or 32 Gm.
1 pound (avoirdupois)	450 Gm.
1 pound	0.4536 kg.
2.2 pounds (imperial or avoirdupois—not apothecaries')	1 kilogram (kg.)
2.6 pounds (apothecaries'— which is not used by nurses)	1 kg.

METRIC SYSTEM

During the latter part of the eighteenth century the French devised the metric system based upon the decimal system and unalterable standards of measurement. Then, in 1875, the International Bureau of Weights and Measures was established in Paris by the International Metric Convention. This Bureau prepared international standards for the participating countries.

The metric units of measurement are the *gram* (weight), *liter* (volume), and *meter* (linear). These basic units can be divided by or multiplied by 10, 100, or 1000. Latin prefixes are used to designate the subdivisions of these units and Greek prefixes are used to designate multiples of these units as shown below for the gram (Gm.).

1 kilogram (kg.)	= 1000.	Gm.
1 hectogram (Hg.)	= 100.	Gm.
1 dekagram (Dg.)	= 10.	Gm.
1 gram (Gm.)	= 1.0	Gm.
1 decigram (dg.)	= 0.1	Gm.
1 centigram (cg.)	= 0.01	Gm.
1 milligram (mg.)	= 0.001	Gm.

The metric system of measurement is used in most of the world. Its use, especially in drug administration, is becoming more prevalent in the United States.

TABLE 6. Additional approximate metric/apothecaries' weight equivalents

METRIC		APOTHECARIES'
	30 or 32 Gm.	1 oz.
	15 or 16 Gm.	4 dr.
	7.5 or 8 Gm.	2 dr.
	6 Gm.	90 to 96 gr.
	5 Gm.	75 to 80 gr.
	4 Gm.	60 to 64 gr. or 1 dr.
	3 Gm.	45 to 48 gr.
	2 Gm.	30 to 32 gr. or 1/2 dr.
	1.5 Gm.	22 1/2 to 24 gr.
1000 mg.	1 Gm.	15 to 16 gr.*
750 mg.	0.75 Gm.	11 1/4 to 12 gr.
600 mg.	0.6 Gm.	9 to 9 3/5 gr. or 10 gr.
500 mg.	0.5 Gm.	7 1/2 to 8 gr.
400 mg.	0.4 Gm.	6 to 6 2/5 gr.
300 mg.	0.3 Gm.	4 1/2 to 4 4/5 gr. or 5 gr.
250 mg.	0.25 Gm.	3 3/4 to 4 gr.
200 mg.	0.2 Gm.	3 to 3 1/5 gr.
150 mg.	0.15 Gm.	2 1/4 to 2 2/5 gr. or 2 1/2 gr.
120 mg.	0.12 Gm.	1 4/5 to 1 9/10 gr. or 2 gr.
100 mg.	0.1 Gm.	1 1/2 to 1 3/5 gr.
75 mg.	0.075 Gm.	1 1/8 to 1 1/5 gr.
60, 64, or 65 mg.	0.06 to 0.065 Gm.	1 gr.
50 mg.	0.05 Gm.	3/4 to 4/5 gr.
40 mg.	0.04 Gm.	3/5 to 16/25 gr.
30 mg.	0.03 Gm.	9/20 to 12/25 gr. or 1/2 gr.
25 mg.	0.025 Gm.	3/8 to 2/5 gr.
20 mg.	0.02 Gm.	3/10 to 8/25 gr. or 1/3 gr.
15 mg.	0.015 Gm.	9/40 to 6/25 gr. or 1/4 gr.
12 mg.	0.012 Gm.	9/50 to 24/125 gr. or 1/5 gr.
10 mg.	0.010 Gm.	3/20 to 4/25 gr. or 1/6 gr.
8 mg.	0.008 Gm.	3/25 to 16/125 gr. or 1/8 gr.
6 mg.	0.006 Gm.	9/100 to 12/125 gr. or 1/10 gr.
5 mg.	0.005 Gm.	3/40 to 2/25 gr. or 1/12 gr.
4 mg.	0.004 Gm.	3/50 to 8/125 gr. or 1/15 to 1/16 gr.
3 mg.	0.003 Gm.	9/200 to 6/125 gr. or 1/20 gr.
2 mg.	0.002 Gm.	3/100 to 4/125 gr. or 1/30 gr.
1.5 mg.	0.0015 Gm.	9/400 to 3/125 gr. or 1/40 gr.
1.2 mg.	0.0012 Gm.	9/500 to 12/625 gr. or 1/50 gr.
1 mg.	0.001 Gm.	3/200 to 2/125 gr. or 1/60, 1/64, or 1/65 gr.

*Often when using both 15 and 16 grains = 1 gram to determine these grain equivalent, the answer is a fraction which is awkward to use. In such instances, a nearly equal, simplified fraction is listed also.

TABLE 6. Additional approximate metric/apothecaries' weight equivalents (continued)

METRIC		APOTHECARIES'
0.8 mg.	0.0008 Gm.	3/250 to 8/625 gr. or 1/80 gr.
0.6 mg.	0.0006 Gm.	9/1000 to 6/625 gr. or 1/100 gr.
0.5 mg.	0.0005 Gm.	1/120, 1/128, or 1/130 gr.
0.4 mg.	0.0004 Gm.	3/500 to 4/625 gr. or 1/150 to 1/160 gr.
0.3 mg.	0.0003 Gm.	9/2000 to 3/625 gr. or 1/200 to 1/210 gr.
0.25 mg.	0.00025 Gm.	3/800 to 1/250 gr.
0.2 mg.	0.0002 Gm.	3/1000 to 2/625 gr. or 1/300 to 1/320 gr.
0.15	0.00015 Gm.	9/4000 to 3/1250 gr. or 1/400 gr.
0.12	0.00012 Gm.	9/5000 to 6/3125 gr. or 1/500 gr.
0.1 mg.	0.001 Gm.	3/2000 to 1/625 gr. or 1/600, 1/640, or 1/650 gr.

TABLE 7. Exact metric/apothecaries' equivalents

12 METRIC	APOTHECARIES'
31.1035 Gm.	1 oz.
1 Gm.	15.432 gr.
0.972 Gm.	15 gr.
0.648 Gm.	10 gr.
0.324 Gm.	5 gr.
0.0648 Gm.	1 gr.
1 ml.	16.23 m.

Gram

The gram, the metric unit of weight used in the pharmaceutical weighing of drugs, is equal to the weight of one milliliter of distilled water at 4°C. The kilogram (1000 Gm.) is the only multiple of the gram used by nurses. It may be used to calculate dosages, fluids, and so forth in terms of kilograms of body weight. The only subdivisions of a gram commonly used are the milligram (0.001 Gm.) and the microgram (0.001 mg.).

Liter

The liter, the metric volume unit which is very frequently used by nurses, is equal to the contents of one decimeter (10 centimeters) cube. The liter was found to be 1000.028 cubic centimeters (cc.) rather than the 1000 cc. intended. A liter does contain 1000 milliliters (ml.), of course. Even though a cubic centimeter is 0.000028 cc. less than a milliliter, in drug administration a cubic centimeter and a milliliter are considered to be equal and are used interchangeably.

Since a gram is equal to the weight of one milliliter of distilled water at 4°C, *1 Gm. = 1 ml.* is an equivalent that may safely be used in the calculation of dosage and solutions problems when needed. This equivalent is an approximate, not an accurate one, when used for such purposes.

Meter

The meter, the metric linear unit of measurement, is 39.37 inches. Centimeters, millimeters, and, occasionally, microns (one thousandth of a millimeter) are the only linear metric measures used by nurses. There are approximately 2.5 centimeters per one inch. The sides of a cubic centimeter (cc.) are approximately 0.4 inch each.

ABBREVIATIONS USED IN DRUG ADMINISTRATION

ABBREVIATION	MEANING	ABBREVIATION	MEANING
a̅a̅	of each	o.d. or q.d.	every day
a.c.	before meals	o.m. or q.a.m.	every morning
ad.	up to	o.n. or q.p.m.	every night
aq.	water	O.S.	left eye
aq. dest. or D.W.	distilled water	os	mouth
		OU	both eyes
b.i.d.	twice a day	oz.	ounce
c̅	with	p.c.	after meals
caps.	capsules	per	by
comp.	compound	per os or p.o.	by mouth
dil.	dilute	p.r.n.	when required
elix.	elixir	q.h.	every hour
ext.	extract	q.2h.	every 2 hours
fld. or fl.	fluid	q.3h.	every 3 hours
Ft.	make	q.4h.	every 4 hours
Gm.	gram	q.i.d.	four times a day
gr.	grain	q.o.d.	every other day
gtt.	drop	q.o.h.	every other hour
H.	by hypodermic	q.s.	quantity sufficient
h. or hr.	hour	R	take
h.s.	hour of sleep	s̅	without
I.M.	intramuscularly	s.c.	subcutaneously
I.V.	intravenously	Sig. or S.	write on label
kg.	kilogram	sol.	solution
M.	mix	s.o.s.	once if necessary
m.	minim	sp.	spirits
mixt. or mist.	mixture	s̅s̅	a half
		stat.	immediately
n., noc. or noct.	night	syr.	syrup
		t.i.d.	three times a day
non rep.	not to be repeated	tr. or tinct.	tincture
O	pint	U.	unit
ol.	oil	ung.	ointment
O.D.	right eye	vin.	wine

APPENDIX C

ARITHMETIC REVIEW

PRETEST IN ARITHMETIC

Which is larger:

1. 1/150 or 1/200?

2. 3/7 or 3/8?

3. 100/1 or 3/2?

4. 0.006 or 0.03?

5. 1:20 or 1:2?

6. 1/10% or 1/5%?

Complete the following:

7. $2/7 + 2/3 =$

8. $1/100 + 1/100 =$

9. $1\ 1/2 + 3/4 =$

10. $1/2 + 1/3 + 1\ 1/4 =$

11. $1/4\% + 1/3\% =$

12. $0.04 + 0.033 =$

13. $1:5 + 4:6 =$

14. $1/100 - 1/150 =$

15. $4/3 - 7/6 =$

16. $1\ 1/2 - 1\ 1/3 =$

17. $0.66 - 0.06 =$

18. $1/1000 \times 1 =$

19. $0.03 \times 2 =$

20. $100/1 \times 5 =$

21. $2/3 \times 1/2 =$

22. $1\ 1/2 \times 1/3 =$

23. $1\ 1/2 \div 1/3 =$

24. $300/150 \div 2 =$

25. $3/4 \div 2/3 =$

26. $1.5 \div 0.1 =$

27. $0.5 \div 3/4 =$

28. $\dfrac{1/3}{1/2} =$

29. $\dfrac{1\ 1/2}{2} =$

Change to decimal fractions:

30. 1/10

31. 2%

32. 15/1

33. 2:50

Change to ratios:

34. 1

35. 75%

36. 1/1000

37. 0.5%

38. 0.125%

Change to percent:

39. 1/300

40. 1/2

41. 1:1000

42. 0.75

43. 2 1/2

Solve for x, the unknown value:

44. $400:1 = 1000:x$

45. $80:16 = 100:x$

46. $15:1000 = x:100$

47. $\dfrac{1}{10,000} : \dfrac{1}{8000} = x:4000$

48. $100:1000 = 1/4:x$

Round off to the nearest hundredth:

49. 0.666 2/3

50. 0.3 1/3

Write these Roman numerals in Arabic numbers:

51. IX =

52. vi =

53. XC =

54. XII =

55. LX =

Write these Arabic numbers in Roman numerals:

56. 4 =

57. 2000 =

58. 6 =

59. 15 =

60. 100 =

Change to °C:

61. 97°F

62. − 40°F

63. 110°F

64. 65°F

65. 105°F

Change to °F:

66. 10°C

67. 40°C

68. − 10°C

69. 32°C

70. 37°C

COMMON FRACTIONS

A *proper fraction* is one in which the numerator is less than the denominator, e.g., 1/2, 3/4, 2/3, 5/6, 1/200.

An *improper fraction* is one in which the numerator is equal to, or greater than, the denominator, e.g., 2/2, 7/5, 300/150.

A *mixed number* is a whole number plus a fraction, e.g., 1 1/3, 2 1/2, 10 2/3, 25 7/8.

A *mixed number* can be changed to an *improper fraction* by multiplying the whole number by the denominator, adding the numerator, and placing the sum over the denominator, e.g., $1\ 1/3 = \dfrac{3 \times 1 + 1}{3} = 4/3$.

An *improper fraction* can be changed to a *whole* or a *mixed number* by dividing the numerator by the denominator, e.g., 7/5 = 7 ÷ 5 = 1 2/7.

A *whole number* has an unexpressed denominator of 1, e.g., 4 = 4/1, 1 = 1/1, 1000 = 1000/1.

A *complex fraction* is one in which the numerator, the denominator, or both, are fractions, e.g.,

$$\frac{1\ 1/2}{2},\ \frac{1/1000}{1},\ \frac{1/3}{1/2},\ \frac{1}{1/100}.$$

To *simplify a complex fraction* divide the numerator by the denominator after reducing either or both, as needed, to a simpler fraction, e.g.,

$$\frac{1\ 1/2}{2} = \frac{3/2}{2} = 3/2 \div 2/1 = 3/2 \times 1/2 = 3/4.$$

To *add common fractions* change fractions to equivalent fractions with the least common denominator, add the numerators, and write this sum over the common denominator. A least common denominator is the smallest number into which all denominators can be divided evenly.

Adding proper fractions:
   1/300 + 1/150 + 1/10 = 1/300 + 2/300 + 30/300 = 33/300 = 11/100

Adding improper fractions:
   1/1 + 4/3 + 9/7 = 21/21 + 28/21 + 27/21 = 76/21 = 3 13/21

Adding mixed numbers:
   1 1/3 + 2 1/2 = 4/3 + 5/2 = 8/6 + 15/6 = 23/6 = 3 5/6

Adding whole numbers and fractions:
  2 + 1/2 = 2/1 + 1/2 = 4/2 + 1/2 = 5/2 = 2 1/2

  To subtract common fractions again reduce to equivalent fractions with the least common denominator, subtract the numerator with the minus sign from the other numerator and place the remainder over the common denominator.

Subtracting proper fractions:
  1/150 − 1/300 = 2/300 − 1/300 = 1/300

Subtracting improper fractions:
  3/2 − 5/4 = 6/4 − 5/4 = 1/4

Subtracting mixed numbers:
  1 1/3 − 1 1/4 = 4/3 − 5/4 = 16/12 − 15/12 = 1/12   *or*

$$4\,3/4 - 2\,1/2 = \quad \begin{matrix} 4\,3/4 \\ -2\,1/2 \\ \hline \end{matrix} = \begin{matrix} 4\,3/4 \\ -2\,2/4 \\ \hline 2\,1/4 \end{matrix} \quad or$$

$$4\,1/2 - 2\,3/4 = \quad \begin{matrix} 4\,1/2 \\ -2\,3/4 \\ \hline \end{matrix} = \begin{matrix} 4\,2/4 \\ -2\,3/4 \\ \hline \end{matrix} = \begin{matrix} 3\,6/4 \\ -2\,3/4 \\ \hline 1\,3/4 \end{matrix}$$

Subtracting whole numbers and fractions:
  5 − 2 1/2 = 5/1 − 5/2 = 10/2 − 5/2 = 5/2 = 2 1/2   *or*

$$5 - 2\,1/2 = \quad \begin{matrix} 5 \\ -2\,1/2 \\ \hline \end{matrix} = \begin{matrix} 4\,2/2 \\ -2\,1/2 \\ \hline 2\,1/2 \end{matrix}$$

  To multiply common fractions multiply the numerators together and the denominators together then reduce the resulting fraction to its lowest terms.

Multiplying proper fractions:
  2/3 × 3/4 = 6/12 = 1/2   *or*   1/100 × 1/2 = 1/2000

Multiplying improper fractions:
  2/1 × 3/2 = 6/2 = 3   *or*   300/150 × 1/1 = 300/150 = 2

Multiplying mixed numbers:
  1 1/3 × 2 1/2 = 4/3 × 5/2 = 20/6 = 3 2/6 = 3 1/3

Multiplying whole numbers by fractions:
  2 × 1/100 = 2/1 = 1/1000 = 2/1000 = 1/500   *or*
  1 × 1/2 = 1/1 × 1/2   *or*   1/200 × 2 = 1/200 × 2/1 = 2/200 = 1/100

To *divide common fractions* invert the divisor and multiply.

Dividing proper fractions:
   2/3 ÷ 3/4 = 2/3 × 4/3 = 8/9   *or*   1/2 ÷ 1/2 = 1/2 × 2/1 = 2/2 = 1

Dividing improper fractions:
   3/2 ÷ 2/1 = 3/2 × 1/2 = 3/4   *or*
   300/150 ÷ 2/1 = 300/150 × 1/2 = 300/300 = 1

Dividing mixed numbers:
   1 1/2 ÷ 2 1/3 = 3/2 ÷ 7/3 = 3/2 × 3/7 = 9/14

Dividing whole numbers and fractions:
   100 ÷ 1/2 = 100/1 ÷ 1/2 = 100/1 × 2/1 = 200   *or*
   1/2 ÷ 100 = 1/2 ÷ 100/1 = 1/2 × 1/100 = 1/200

To compare sizes of fractions is often very important for nurses.

   If numerators are the same the fraction with the smaller denominator represents the larger value, e.g., 1/2 is larger than 1/4, and 1/150 is larger than 1/300. Fractions with different denominators can be compared by changing to the same denominator, e.g., 1/150 and 1/300 to 2/300 and 1/300, or 1/2 and 1/4 to 2/4 and 1/4.

   If denominators are the same the fraction with the larger numerator represents the larger value, e.g., 2/300 is larger than 1/300.

DECIMAL FRACTIONS

A decimal fraction is a fraction whose denominator is any power of ten and which may be expressed in decimal form.

   Changing common fractions to decimal fractions is done by dividing the numerator by the denominator, e.g.,

$$1/2 = 2\overline{)1.0}^{\,0.5} \quad or \quad 1/200 = 200\overline{)1.000}^{\,0.005}$$

   Changing decimal fractions to common fractions is done more easily but great caution should be taken in determining the correct denominator, as shown below.

0.1	= 1/10	or one-tenth
0.01	= 1/100	or one-hundredth
0.001	= 1/1000	or one-thousandth
0.0001	= 1/10,000	or one ten-thousandth

```
0.741  = 741/1000
0.3    = 3/10
0.4276 = 4276/10,000
0.005  = 5/1000
```

To *add and subtract decimals* place the decimal points in vertical alignment.

Adding decimals:

$$0.0004 + 0.006 = \begin{array}{r} 0.0004 \\ 0.0060 \\ \hline 0.0064 \end{array}$$

Subtracting decimals:

$$0.06 - 0.004 = \begin{array}{r} 0.060 \\ 0.004 \\ \hline 0.056 \end{array}$$

To *multiply decimals* first multiply as with whole numbers; then, count off from the right in the product as many decimal places as there are in both the multiplier and the multiplicand.

Multiplying decimals:

$$1.25 \times 0.75 = \begin{array}{r} 1.25 \\ 0.75 \\ \hline 625 \\ 875 \\ \hline 0.9375 \end{array}$$

To *divide decimals* divide as with whole numbers *after* converting the divisor to a whole number by moving the decimal point to the far right and after moving the decimal point in the dividend the same number of places to the right, adding zeros as necessary.

Dividing decimals:

$$1.125 \div 0.75 = 0.75\overline{)1.125} = \begin{array}{r} 1.5 \\ 75\overline{)112.5} \\ 75 \\ \hline 375 \\ 375 \\ \hline \end{array}$$

or

$$0.6 \div 0.03 = 0.03\overline{)0.6} = \begin{array}{r} 20. \\ 3\overline{)60.} \\ 60 \\ \hline \end{array}$$

PERCENTAGE

A *percent* is a part of 100 equal parts. It is a fraction with a denominator of 100.

To change percent to a common fraction write the percent as the numerator and replace the % symbol with 100 as the denominator of the fraction, as shown below.

$$5\% = 5/100 = 1/20$$

$$1/10\% = \frac{1/10}{100} = 1/10 \div 100/1 = 1/10 \times 1/100 = 1/1000$$

$$0.2\% = \frac{2/10}{100} = 2/10 \div 100/1 = 2/10 \times 1/100 = 2/1000 = 1/500$$

To change common fractions to percent divide the numerator by the denominator and *multiply* the quotient by 100 (move decimal point 2 places to the right), as shown below.

$$1/8 = 8\overline{)1.000}^{\ 0.125} = 0.125 \times 100 = 12.5\%$$

$$3/5 = 5\overline{)3.0}^{\ 0.6} = 0.6 \times 100 = 60\%$$

$$1/1000 = 1000\overline{)1.000}^{\ 0.001} = 0.001 \times 100 = 0.1\%$$

To change percent to decimal fractions drop the percent sign and *divide* by 100 (move decimal point 2 places to the left), as shown below.

$$12.5\% = 0.125$$
$$60\% = 0.6$$
$$0.1\% = 0.001$$

RATIO AND PROPORTION

A ratio is the same as a fraction. *A proportion* consists of two ratios or fractions that are equal in value. The ratio 1:20 means that in every 20 parts of a substance such as a solvent, there is one equal part of another substance such as a solute. The ratio 1:20 equals the ratio 5:100 and these two ratios have the same relative values or are in proportion, e.g., 1:20 = 5:100.

The first and last terms of a proportion are called *the extremes*; the second and third terms, *the means*. The product of the means equals the product of the extremes. When any three of the four terms are known, the fourth term can be calculated.

An *unknown mean* is found by dividing the product of the extremes by the known mean, as shown below.

$$4:20 = x:25 \quad \text{or} \quad 4:x = 5:25$$
$$20\,x = 100 \qquad\qquad 5\,x = 100$$
$$\qquad\qquad\qquad\qquad x = 20$$

$$\frac{20\,x}{20} = \frac{100}{20}$$

$$x = 5$$

An *unknown extreme* is found by dividing the product of the means by the known extreme, as follows:

$$x:20 = 5:25 \quad \text{or} \quad 4:20 = 5:x$$
$$25\,x = 100 \qquad\qquad 4\,x = 100$$
$$\qquad\qquad\qquad\qquad x = 25$$

$$\frac{25\,x}{25} = \frac{100}{25}$$

$$x = 4$$

Actually this is the same as saying that after multiplying the means and extremes, one divides both sides of the resulting equation by the number which precedes the x, the unknown value.

A more detailed explanation of the use of ratio and proportion is given in the text of this workbook.

CENTIGRADE/FAHRENHEIT CONVERSIONS

There are two thermal scales used in the United States, the degrees of Fahrenheit (°F) and the degrees of Centigrade (°C), or Celcius scales. Most of the world uses only the Celcius scale. On the Fahrenheit scale freezing is 32°F and boiling is 212°F. On the Celcius or Centigrade scale freezing is 0°C and boiling is 100°C (Fig. 19). Formulas for conversion are shown below.

To convert °F to °C, first subtract 32° from the °F, then multiply times 5/9.

$$°C = (°F - 32)\, 5/9$$

212 °F = ? °C   32 °F = ? °C
°C = (212 − 32)5/9   °C = (32 − 32)5/9
°C = 180 × 5/9   °C = 0 × 5/9
°C = 100°   °C = 0°

To convert °C to °F, first multiply the number of °C times 9/5, then add 32°C.

$$°F = (°C × 9/5) + 32$$

126

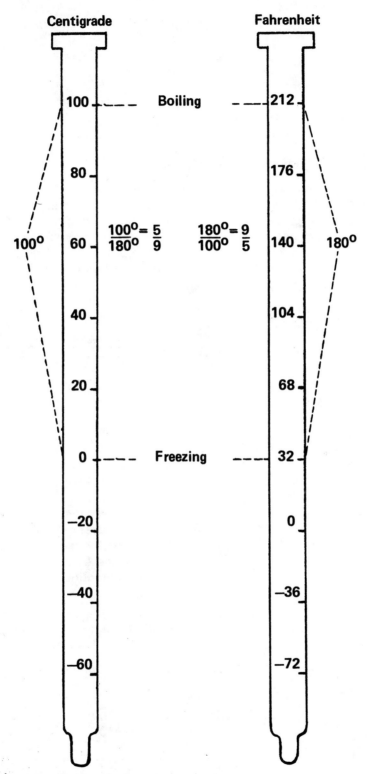

FIGURE 19. Centigrade and Fahrenheit thermometers.

$100°C = ?°F$

$°F = (100 \times 9/5) + 32$

$°F = 180 + 32$

$°F = 212°$

$98°F = ?°C$

$°C = (98 - 32)5/9$

$°C = 66 \times 5/9$

$°C = 36.67°$

$0°C = ?°F$

$°F = (0 \times 9/5) + 32$

$°F = 0 + 32$

$°F = 32°$

$40°C = ?°F$

$°F = (40 \times 9/5) + 32$

$°F = 72 + 32$

$°F = 104°$

ROMAN AND ARABIC NUMERALS

Currently there are two systems of counting: Arabic numbers and Roman numerals. The Arabic system is used in the ordering and calculations of medication dosages. The Arabic numerals, or digits, are 1, 2, 3, 4, 5, 6, 7, 8, 9, and 0. It can be used with whole numbers, common fractions, decimal fractions, percentages, and ratios and proportions. This system is used with both metric and household measures. The decimal place values of Arabic numbers are shown in Table 8.

TABLE 8. Place values of arabic numbers

WHOLE NUMBERS		DECIMAL FRACTIONS	
Millions	1,000,000		
Hundred thousands	100,000		
Ten thousands	10,000		
Thousands	1,000		
Hundreds	100		
Tens	10		
Units	1		
No value	0.0	No value	
	0.1	Tenths	
	0.01	Hundreths	
	0.001	Thousandths	
	0.0001	Ten thousandths	
	0.00001	Hundred thousandths	
	0.000001	Millionths	

Sometimes Roman numerals are used with the apothecaries' system to prescribe or calculate drug dosages. Seven capital letters may be used to express Roman numerals.

Roman numerals	Arabic numbers
I	1
V	5
X	10
L	50
C	100
D	500
M	1,000

Frequently lower case numerals are used to prescribe the amount of drugs or solutions, especially small amounts.

Roman numerals	Arabic numbers
i or $\dot{\text{i}}$	1
v or $\bar{\text{v}}$	5
x or $\bar{\text{x}}$	10

A combination of Roman numerals are used to indicate other numbers. When a numeral of lesser value precedes a numeral of greater value, subtract the one of lesser value from the one of greater value. Only one numeral is ever subtracted.

Roman numerals	Arabic numbers
IV or $\dot{\text{iv}}$	4
IX or $\dot{\text{ix}}$	9
XL	40

When a numeral of lesser value follows one of greater value, add the one of lesser value to the one of greater value. Only three numerals are ever added.

Roman numerals	Arabic numbers
ii or ii	2
VI or vi	6
XV or XV	15
XX or XX	20
XXV or xxv	25
XXX or xxx	30

Sometimes the symbol ss, used to express one-half, is used with Roman numerals.

Roman numerals	Arabic numbers
$\overline{\text{ss}}$ or $\overset{..}{\overline{\text{ss}}}$ or ss	1/2
$\overline{\text{iss}}$ or $\overset{...}{\overline{\text{iss}}}$ or iss	1 1/2
$\overline{\text{iiss}}$ or $\overset{....}{\overline{\text{iiss}}}$ or iiss	2 1/2
$\overline{\text{viiss}}$ or $\overset{....}{\overline{\text{viiss}}}$ or viss	7 1/2

Practice Problems

1. $\dfrac{1\,1/2}{2} =$

2. $\dfrac{1\,3/4}{2} =$

3. $\dfrac{2\,1/4}{3} =$

4. $\dfrac{1/3}{1} =$

5. $\dfrac{1\,1/3}{2} =$

Adding Common Fractions

6. $1/150 + 1/300 =$

7. $1\,1/2 + 3/4 =$

8. $4/3 + 3/2 =$

9. $1\,1/2 + 2\,1/3 =$

10. $1/1000 + 1/1 =$

11. $2/1 + 1/2 =$

12. $1/100 + 1/200 =$

13. $4/3 + 5/4 =$

14. $1\,1/4 + 1\,1/5 =$

15. $3 + 1/300 =$

Subtracting Common Fractions

16. $1/150 - 1/200 =$

17. $4/3 - 1/2 =$

18. $1\,1/2 - 1\,1/4 =$

19. $3 - 1\,1/3 =$

20. $1/1000 - 1/2000 =$

21. $5/4 - 1/3 =$

22. $3\,1/2 - 2\,1/3 =$

23. $100 - 33\,1/3 =$

24. $1000 - 666\,2/3 =$

25. $2 - 1\,1/3 =$

Multiplying Common Fractions

26. $1/3 \times 1/2 =$

27. $3/2 = 5/4 =$

28. $2\,1/3 \times 1\,1/2 =$

29. $2 \times 1/1000 =$

30. $1/8000 \times 1/1000 =$

31. $1/10,000 \times 100 =$

32. $1/12,000 \times 1 =$

33. $1/8 \times 1\,1/4 =$

34. $2/100 = 3000/1 =$

35. $1000 \times 1\,1/2 =$

36. $1 \times 1/120 =$

37. $1/4 \times 32 =$

38. $60 \times 1\,1/2 =$

39. $64 \times 1\,1/2 =$

40. $1/10,000 \times 1000 =$

41. $1/8 \times 30 =$

42. $1/8 \times 32 =$

43. $2/1 \times 10,000/1 =$

44. $1/8 \times x =$

45. $1/1 \times x =$

46. $1 \times 1/100 =$

47. $1/200 \times x =$

48. $64 \times 1/3 =$

49. $60 \times 1/3 =$

50. $5/100 \times 3000/1 =$

Dividing Common Fractions

51. $2/3 \div 3/4 =$

52. $1/4 \div 1/4 =$

53. $\dfrac{3/4}{1/2} =$

54. $300/150 \div 2/1 =$

55. $\dfrac{3/2}{2/1} =$

56. $1\,1/4 \div 2\,1/3 =$

57. $1000 \div 1/3 =$

58. $1000/12,000 \div 1/8000 =$

59. $4 \div 40/1 =$

60. $1/8 \div 1/12,000 =$

61. $\dfrac{1\,1/4}{2} =$

62. $1/200 \div 1/100 =$

63. $1000/10,000 \div 1/1000 =$

64. $\dfrac{1\,1/2}{2} =$

65. $1/200 \div 1/150 =$

66. $1000/12,000 \div 1/1 =$

67. $1/2 \div 1 =$

68. $100 \div 9/10 =$

69. $30 \div 1/8 =$

70. $32 \div 1/8 =$

71. $1/120 \div 1/60 =$

72. $64 \div 3/4 =$

73. $60 \div 3/4 =$

74. $1/150 \div 1/2 =$

75. $1\,2/3 \div 2 =$

Comparing Sizes of Fractions

WHICH IS SMALLER:

76. 1/2 or 1/3?

77. 1/150 or 1/200?

78. 1/10,000 or 1/8000?

79. 1/300 or 1/150?

80. 2/300 or 1/300?

81. 2/4 or 4/2?

82. 1/1 or 1/2?

83. 1000/1 or 500/1?

84. 1/64 or 1/60?

85. 2/1 or 4/3?

Changing Common Fractions to Decimal Fractions

86. $1/2 =$

87. 1/200 =

88. 5/100 =

89. 1/100 =

90. 2/100 =

91. 3/4 =

92. 2/3 =

93. 1/10,000 =

94. 1/8 =

95. 2 1/4 =

Changing Decimal Fractions to Common Fractions

96. 0.0001 =

97. 0.03 =

98. 0.50 =

99. 0.01 =

100. 0.005 =

101. 0.500 =

102. 0.27 =

103. 0.6 =

104. 1.125 =

105. 0.25 =

Adding Decimals

106. 0.004 + 0.006 =

107. 0.5 + 0.25 =

108. 0.05 + 0.5 =

109. 0.003 + 0.0006 =

110. 1.33 + 0.050 =

Subtracting Decimals

111. 0.06 − 0.004 =

112. 0.5 − 0.25 =

113. 0.004 − 0.0005 =

114. 0.25 − 0.125 =

115. 0.006 − 0.003 =

Multiplying Decimals

116. 1.25 × 0.75 =

117. 0.5 × 0.5 =

118. 0.1 × 0.01 =

119. 0.008 × 1.0 =

120. 0.001 × 1.5 =

Dividing Decimals

121. 1.25 ÷ 75 =

122. 0.6 ÷ 0.03 =

123. 0.1 ÷ 0.01 =

124. 0.5 ÷ 0.5 =

125. 0.1 ÷ 0.005 =

Changing Percents to Common Fractions

126. 0.2% =

127. 1/10% =

128. 15% =

129. 100% =

130. 0.01% =

Changing Common Fractions to Percents

131. 1/8 =

132. 1/10,000 =

133. 1 1/2 =

134. 1/100 =

135. 1/500 =

Changing Percents to Decimal Fractions

136. 0.1% =

137. 2% =

138. 50% =

139. 0.0125% =

140. 100% =

Determining Unknown Mean in Ratio and Proportion

141. $5:100 = x:60$

142. $2:100 = x:1000$

143. $10:x = 0.5:10,000$

144. $16:x = 40:16$

145. $2/100:1/2 = x:3000$

146. $1000:x = 125:1$

147. $0.5:x = 0.3:1$

148. $300,000:x = 150,000:5$

149. $0.5:x = 0.25:1$

150. $1/12,000:1/8000 = x:1000$

Determining Unknown Extreme in Ratio and Proportion

151. $16:1000 = 1:x$

152. $1:60 = 1\ 1/2:x$

153. $60:1 = 15:x$

154. $x:100 = 30:600$

155. $1/10,000:1/1 = 30:x$

156. $80:16 = 18:x$

157. $125:1 = 1000:x$

158. $300,000:1 = 3,000,000:x$

159. $0.3:1 = 0.5:x$

160. $1/150:1 = 1/200:x$

Converting °F to °C

161. 212 °F =

162. 32 °F =

163. 82 °F =

164. 0 °F =

165. 60 °F =

Converting °C to °F

166. 0 °C =

167. 100 °C =

168. 20 °C =

169. 35 °C =

170. 40 °C =

Changing Roman Numerals to Arabic Numbers

171. IXX =

172. vii =

173. XC =

174. xvi =

175. LX =

Changing Arabic Numbers to Roman Numerals

176. 4 =

177. 12 =

178. 8 =

179. 1,000 =

180. 150 =

REVIEW PROBLEMS

Which is larger:

1. 1/300 or 1/150?

2. 0.5% or 1/5%?

3. 1/12,000 or 1/8000?

4. 0.006 or 0.03?

5. 0.5 or 0.25?

Change to decimal fractions:

6. 8%

7. 1:100

8. 1/25

Change to ratios:

9. 2

10. 1/10,000

11. 0.2%

Change to percent:

12. 1:20

13. 1/150

14. 1:10,000

Round off the the nearest thousandth:

15. 0.333 1/3

16. 0.6 2/3

17. 1 1/3

Complete the following:

18. 1/300 + 1/150 =

19. 2/3 + 3/2 =

20. 0.025 ÷ 1000 =

21. 0.002 ÷ 0.004 =

22. $\dfrac{1\ 2/3}{2} =$

23. 1/4 ÷ 1/8000 =

24. 4/2 × 3/4 =

25. 0.5 ÷ 0.3 =

26. 10 ÷ 0.05 =

27. 3/2 ÷ 1/2 =

28. 2 − 0.05 =

29. 1 3/4 × 0.05 =

30. $\dfrac{2/3}{1}$ =

31. 60 × 1/3 =

32. 500 − 1/3 =

33. 1.5 ÷ 0.25 =

34. 1000 − 666 2/3 =

35. 1000 × 0.05 =

36. 0.5 × 1/200 =

37. 1 1/3 + 1/4 =

38. 0.005 ÷ 1000 =

39. 1/150 − 1/300 =

40. 1/10,000 × 500 =

Solve for x, the unknown value:

41. 15:1 = x:0.5

42. 1000:1 = 0.025:x

43. 80:16 = 30:x

44. 1:60 = x:32

45. 1/3:1 = x:30

46. 0.5:1 = 10:x

47. 1/12,000:1/8000 = x:3000

48. 200,000:1 = 1,000,000:x

49. 1:1000 = 0.5:x

50. 0.004:1 = 0.002:x

Change to Arabic numbers:

51. $\dot{\text{iv}}$ =

52. $\overset{...}{\text{iss}}$ =

53. XII =

54. ii =

55. M =

56. XXX =

57. xv =

58. $\overset{....}{\text{viiss}}$ =

59. CXX =

60. XV =

Change to Roman numerals:

61. 1 1/2 =

62. 30 =

63. 1000 =

64. 7 1/2 =

65. 15 =

66. 90 =

67. 4 =

68. 60 =

69. 400 =

70. 2500 =

Convert °F to °C:

71. 98.6 °F =

72. 200 °F =

135

73. $-50\ °F =$

74. $10\ °F =$

75. $68\ °F =$

Convert °C to °F:

76. $38\ °C =$

77. $43\ °C =$

78. $10\ °C =$

79. $34\ °C =$

80. $-10\ °C =$

POST-TEST

1. Which is larger, 1/150 or 1/300?

2. $2/3 + 1/4 =$

3. Change 1/100 to a decimal fraction

4. Change 0.125% to a ratio

5. Change 1:1000 to a percent

6. Round off 0.66 to the nearest tenth

7. Solve for x when $60:1 = x:0.50$

8. Convert 98 °F to °C

9. Change IX to an Arabic number

10. $1\ 1/2 \div 1/2 =$

11. $1/60 \times 4 =$

12. Which is smaller, 0.006 or 0.03?

13. Change 3% to a ratio

14. Solve for x when $2x = 300/150$

15. Convert 9 °C to °F

16. Change 7 1/2 to a Roman numeral

17. $0.33 - 0.033 =$

18. Solve for x when $200,000:2 = 300,000:x$

19. $8\ 1/3 \times 15 =$

20. Change 7 1/2 to a percent

21. Solve for x when $125:5 = 0.25:x$

22. Solve for x when $1:1000 = 0.005:x$

23. Change 5% to a decimal fraction

24. Solve for x when $0.25:5 = 0.3:x$

25. $1500 \div 4 =$

26. Solve for x when $1/64:1 = x:32$

27. Change 0.667 to a percent

28. $\dfrac{0.3 \times 500}{1.7} =$

29. $\dfrac{8}{8 + 12} \times 500 =$

30. Solve for x when $1:64 = 1\ 1/2:x$

31. Which is larger, 1/10% or 1/20%?

32. Change 50% to a ratio

33. Solve for x when $1:15 = 8\ 1/3:x$

34. Change 0.5% to a ratio

35. $3000 \div 24 =$

36. Round off 0.666 2/3 to the nearest hundredth

37. Solve for x when $1/60:1 = x:2$

38. Which is larger, 1/200, 1/150, or 1/120?

39. Change 2:1000 to a decimal fraction

40. Solve for x when $4:1 = x:2$

41. Which is smaller, 1:1000 or 1:100?

42. Solve for x when $0.25:1 = 0.5:x$

43. Solve for x when $15:1 = x:0.3$

44. Which is larger, 1:1000 or 1:100?

45. Change 1/150 to a percent.

46. Solve for x when $0.01:1 = x:5$

47. Solve for x when $2.2:1 = 18:x$

48. $\dfrac{0.44 \times 0.5}{1.7} =$

49. Solve for x when $80:1 = x:1.3$

50. Solve for x when $100:16 = 40:x$

ARITHMETIC ANSWERS

Pretest in Arithmetic

1. 1/150
2. 3/7
3. 100/1
4. 0.03
5. 1:2
6. 1/5%
7. 20/21
8. 1/50
9. 2 1/4
10. 2 1/12
11. 7/12%
12. 0.073
13. 13/15
14. 1/300
15. 1/6
16. 1/6
17. 0.60
18. 1/1000
19. 0.06
20. 500
21. 1/3
22. 1/2
23. 4 1/2
24. 1
25. 1 1/8
26. 15
27. 2/3 or 0.67
28. 2/3
29. 3/4
30. 0.1
31. 0.02
32. 15.0
33. 0.04
34. 1:1
35. 75:100 or 3:4
36. 1:1000
37. 5:1000 or 1:200
38. 125:100,000 = 1:800
39. 1/3% or 0.3%
40. 50%
41. 1/10% or 0.1%
42. 75%
43. 250%
44. 2 1/2
45. 20
46. 1 1/2
47. 3200
48. 2 1/2
49. 0.67
50. 0.33
51. 9
52. 6
53. 90
54. 12
55. 60
56. iv
57. MM
58. vi
59. xv
60. C

61. $(97 - 32)5/9 = 65 \times 5/9 = \dfrac{325}{9} = 36.11°C$

62. $(-40 - 32)5/9 = -72 \times 5/9 = \dfrac{-360}{9} = -40°C$

63. $(110 - 32)5/9 = 78 \times 5/9 = \dfrac{390}{9} = 43.33°C$

64. $(65 - 32)5/9 = 33 \times 5/9 = \dfrac{165}{9} = 18.33°C$

65. $(105 - 32)5/9 = 73 \times 5/9 = \dfrac{365}{9} = 40.56°C$

66. $(10 \times 9/5) + 32 = \dfrac{90}{5} + 32 = 18 + 32 = 50°F$

67. $(40 \times 9/5) + 32 = \dfrac{360}{5} + 32 = 72 + 32 = 104°F$

68. $(-10 \times 9/5) + 32 = \dfrac{-90}{5} + 32 = -18 + 32 = 14°F$

69. $(32 \times 9/5) + 32 = \dfrac{288}{5} + 32 = 57.6 + 32 = 89.6°F$

70. $(37 - 9/5) + 32 = \dfrac{333}{5} + 32 = 66.6 + 32 = 98.6°F$

Practice Problems

1.	3/4	24.	333 1/3	47.	1/200 x
2.	7/8	25.	2/3	48.	21 1/3
3.	3/4	26.	1/6	49.	20
4.	1/3	27.	1 7/8	50.	150
5.	2/3	28.	3 1/2	51.	8/9
6.	1/100	29.	1/500	52.	1
7.	2 1/4	30.	1/8,000,000	53.	1 1/2
8.	2 5/6	31.	1/100	54.	1
9.	3 5/6	32.	1/12,000	55.	3/4
10.	1 1/1000	33.	5/32	56.	15/28
11.	2 1/2	34.	60	57.	3000
12.	3/200	35.	1500	58.	666 2/3
13.	2 7/12	36.	1/120	59.	1/10
14.	2 9/20	37.	8	60.	1500
15.	3 1/300	38.	90	61.	5/8
16.	1/600	39.	96	62.	1/2
17.	5/6	40.	1/10	63.	100
18.	1/4	41.	3 3/4	64.	3/4
19.	1 2/3	42.	4	65.	3/4
20.	1/2000	43.	20,000	66.	1/12
21.	11/12	44.	1/8 x	67.	1/2
22.	1 1/6	45.	1 x or x	68.	111 1/9
23.	66 2/3	46.	1/100	69.	240

70.	256	
71.	1/2	
72.	85 1/3	
73.	80	
74.	1/75	
75.	5/6	
76.	1/3	
77.	1/200	
78.	1/10,000	
79.	1/300	
80.	1/300	
81.	2/4	
82.	1/2	
83.	500/1	
84.	1/64	
85.	4/3	
86.	0.5	
87.	0.005	
88.	0.05	
89.	0.01	
90.	0.02	
91.	0.75	
92.	0.6 2/3	
93.	0.0001	
94.	0.125	
95.	2.25	
96.	1/10,000	
97.	3/100	
98.	1/2	
99.	1/100	
100.	1/200	
101.	1/2	
102.	27/100	
103.	3/5	
104.	1 1/8	
105.	1/4	
106.	0.01	
107.	0.75	
108.	0.55	
109.	0.0036	
110.	1.38	
111.	0.056	
112.	0.25	
113.	0.0035	
114.	0.125	
115.	0.003	
116.	0.9375	
117.	0.25	

118.	0.001
119.	0.008
120.	0.0015
121.	0.01 2/3
122.	20
123.	10
124.	1
125.	20
126.	1/500
127.	1/1000
128.	3/20
129.	1/1
130.	1/10,000
131.	12.5%
132.	0.01%
133.	150%
134.	1%
135.	0.2%
136.	0.001
137.	0.02
138.	0.5
139.	0.000125
140.	1.0
141.	3
142.	20
143.	200,000
144.	6.4
145.	120
146.	8
147.	1 2/3
148.	10
149.	2
150.	666 2/3
151.	62 1/2
152.	90
153.	1/4
154.	5
155.	300,000
156.	3 3/5
157.	8
158.	10
159.	1 2/3
160.	3/4
161.	$(212 - 32)5/9$
	$= 180 \times 5/9$
	$= 100°C$
162.	0°C
163.	27.78°C

164.	– 17.78°C
165.	15.56°C
166.	$(0°C \times 9/5 + 32$
	$= 0 + 32$
	$= 32°F$
167.	212°F
168.	68°F
169.	95°F
170.	104°F
171.	19
172.	7
173.	90
174.	16
175.	60
176.	$\overline{\text{iv}}$
177.	$\overset{\cdot\cdot}{\text{xii}}$
178.	$\overset{\cdot\cdot\cdot}{\text{viii}}$
179.	M
180.	CL

Review Problems

1.	1/150
2.	0.5%
3.	1/8000
4.	0.03
5.	0.5
6.	0.08
7.	0.01
8.	0.04
9.	2:1
10.	1:10,000
11.	2:1000 or 1:500
12.	5%
13.	0.6 2/3%
14.	0.01%
15.	0.333
16.	0.667
17.	1.333
18.	1/100
19.	2 1/6
20.	0.000025
21.	0.5
22.	5/6
23.	2,000
24.	1 1/2
25.	1 2/3

26.	200	41.	7.5	56.	30
27.	3	42.	0.000025	57.	15
28.	1.95	43.	6	58.	7 1/2
29.	7/80 or 0.0875	44.	8/15	59.	120
30.	2/3	45.	10	60.	15.
31.	20	46.	20	61.	$\overline{\text{iss}}$
32.	499 2/3	47.	2000	62.	xxx
33.	6	48.	5	63.	M
34.	333 1/3	49.	500	64.	$\overline{\text{viiss}}$
35.	50	50.	0.5	65.	xv
36.	1/400	51.	4	66.	XC
37.	1 7/12	52.	1 1/2	67.	iv
38.	0.000005	53.	12	68.	LX
39.	1/300	54.	2	69.	CD
40.	1/20	55.	1,000	70.	MMD

71. $(98.6 - 32)\dfrac{5}{9} = 66.6 \times \dfrac{5}{9} = \dfrac{333}{9} = 37°C$

72. $(200 - 32)\dfrac{5}{9} = 168 \times \dfrac{5}{9} = \dfrac{840}{9} = 93.3°C$

73. $(-50 - 32)\dfrac{5}{9} = -82 \times \dfrac{5}{9} = \dfrac{-410}{9} = -45.56°C$

74. $(10 - 32)\dfrac{5}{9} = -22 \times \dfrac{5}{9} = \dfrac{-110}{9} = -12.2°C$

75. $(68 - 32)\dfrac{5}{9} = 36 \times \dfrac{5}{9} = \dfrac{180}{9} = 20°C$

76. $\left(38 \times \dfrac{9}{5}\right) + 32 = \dfrac{342}{5} + 32 = 68.4 + 32 = 100.4°F$

77. $\left(43 \times \dfrac{9}{5}\right) + 32 = \dfrac{387}{5} + 32 = 77.4 + 32 = 109.4°F$

78. $\left(10 \times \dfrac{9}{5}\right) + 32 = \dfrac{90}{5} + 32 = 18 + 32 = 50°F$

79. $\left(34 \times \dfrac{9}{5}\right) + 32 = \dfrac{306}{5} + 32 = 61.2 + 32 = 93.2°F$

80. $\left(-10 \times \dfrac{9}{5}\right) + 32 = \dfrac{-90}{5} + 32 = -18 + 32 = 14°F$

Post-Test

1. 1/150 is twice as large as 1/300.
2. 2/3 + 1/4 = 8/12 + 3/12 = 11/12.
3. 0.01.
4. 125:100,000 = 1:800.
5. 1:1000 = 0.1:100 = 0.1%.
6. 0.7
7. 60:1 = x:0.5; 1 x = 60 × 0.5; x = 30.

8. $(98 - 32)\dfrac{5}{9} = 66 \times \dfrac{5}{9} = \dfrac{330}{9} = 36.7C$

9. 9

10. $1\ 1/2 \div 1/2 = 3/2 \times 2/1 = 6/2 = 3.$

11. $1/60 \times 4 = 1/60 \times 4/1 = 4/60 = 1/15.$

12. 0.006 is 1/5 of 0.03.

13. 3:100

14. $2x = \dfrac{300}{150}; \dfrac{2x}{2} = \dfrac{300}{150} \div \dfrac{2}{1}; x = \dfrac{300}{150} \times \dfrac{1}{2}; x = \dfrac{300}{300} = 1.$

15. $(9 \times 9/5) + 32 = \dfrac{81}{5} + 32 = 16.2 + 32 = 48.2\ F$

16. v̈iïss

17. $0.330 - 0.033 = 0.297$

18. $200,000:2 = 300,000:x; 200,000\, x = 600,000; x = \dfrac{600,000}{200,000} = 3.$

19. $8\ 1/3 \times 15 = 25/3 \times 15/1 = 25/1 \times 5/1 = 125.$

20. $\dfrac{7.5}{100} = 0.075.$

21. $125:5 = 0.25:x; 125\,x = 0.25 \times 5; 125\,x = 1.25; x = 1.25 \div 125; x = 0.01.$

22. $1:1000 = 0.005:x; 1\,x = 1000 \times 0.005; x = 5.$

23. $5\% = \dfrac{5}{100} = 0.05.$

24. $0.25:5 = 0.3:x; 0.25\,x = 1.5; x = 1.5 \div 0.25; x = 6.$

25. $1500 \div 4 = \dfrac{1500}{1} \times \dfrac{1}{4} = \dfrac{1500}{4} = 375.$

26. $\dfrac{1}{64}:1 = x:32; 1\,x = \dfrac{1}{64} \times \dfrac{32}{1}; x = \dfrac{32}{64}; x = \dfrac{1}{2}.$

27. $0.667 \times 100 = 66.7\%.$

28. $\dfrac{0.3 \times 500}{1.7} = \dfrac{150}{1.7} = 88.24$

29. $\dfrac{8}{8 + 12} \times 500 = \dfrac{8}{20} \times \dfrac{500}{1} = \dfrac{8}{1} \times \dfrac{25}{1} = 200$ or

    $\dfrac{8}{20} \times \dfrac{500}{1} = \dfrac{2}{5} \times \dfrac{500}{1} = \dfrac{2}{1} \times \dfrac{100}{1} = 200.$

30. $1:64 = 1\dfrac{1}{2}:x; 1\,x = \dfrac{64}{1} \times \dfrac{3}{2}; x = \dfrac{32}{1} \times \dfrac{3}{1}; x = 96.$

31. 1/10% is twice as large as 1/20% (0.0010 vs. 0.0005).

32. 50:100 or 1:2

33. $1:15 = 8\dfrac{1}{3}:x; 1\,x = \dfrac{15}{1} \times \dfrac{25}{3}; x = \dfrac{375}{3}; x = 125.$

34. 0.5:100 or 5:1000 or 1:200.

35. $\dfrac{300}{24} \div 24 = \dfrac{3000}{1} \times \dfrac{1}{24} = \dfrac{3000}{24} = 125.$

36. 0.67

37. $\dfrac{1}{60}:1 = x:2; 1\,x = \dfrac{1}{60} \times \dfrac{2}{1}; x = \dfrac{2}{60}; x = \dfrac{1}{30}.$

38. 1/120 is larger than 1/150; 1/150 is larger than 1/200.
39. $2 \div 100 = 0.002$.
40. $4:1 = x:2; 1x = 8$.
41. 1:1000 is one-tenth of 1:100.
42. $0.25:1 = 0.5:x; 0.25x = 0.5; x = 0.5 \div 0.25; x = 2$.
43. $15:1 = x:0.3; 1x = 15 \times 0.3; x = 4.5$.
44. 1:100 is ten times as large as 1:1000.
45. $1/150 = 1 \div 150 = 0.006 \ 2/3 = 0.7\%$.
46. $0.01:1 = x:5; 1x = 0.01 \times 5; x = 0.05$.
47. $2.2:1 = 18:x; 2.2x = 18; x = 18 \div 2.2; x = 8.18$.
48. $\dfrac{0.44 \times 0.5}{1.7} = \dfrac{0.22}{1.7} = 0.129$.
49. $80:1 \ x:1.3; 1x = 1.3 \times 80; x = 104$.
50. $100:16 = 40:x; 100x = 40 \times 16; 100x = 640; x = 6.4$.

APPENDIX D

ANSWERS

The answers are provided for use by students and instructors. Sometimes more than one correct answer is given. Depending upon the equivalents or methods of calculation used, additional correct answers (which are not shown here) may result.

CHAPTER 1
PRACTICE PROBLEMS

1. 50 mg. (15 gr. = 1000 mg.) or 45, 48, or 48.75 mg. (1 gr. = 60, 64, or 65 mg.)
2. 5 gr. (1 gr. = 60 mg.) or 4.5 gr. (15 gr. = 1 Gm.)
3. 600 mg. (1000 mg. = 1 Gm.)
4. 1/300 gr. (1 gr. = 60 mg.) or 3/1000 or 1/333 (15 gr. = 1000 mg.)
5. 0.75 Gm. (1000 mg. = 1 Gm.)
6. 5 mg. (1000 mg. = 1 Gm.)
7. 0.5 Gm. (15 gr. = 1 Gm.)
8. 8 ml. (1 dr. = 4 ml.)
9. 0.1 Gm. (15 gr. = 1 Gm.)
10. 300–333 mg. (15 or 16 gr. = 1 Gm. = 1000 mg.)
11. 15 or 16 ml. (2 Tbsp. = 1 oz. or 30–32 ml.)
12. 30 mg. (1 Gm. = 1000 mg.)
13. 59.09 or 59.1 kg.
14. 10 ml.
15. 8 ml.
16. 5 fl. dr.

CHAPTER 2
PRACTICE PROBLEMS

1. 1/2 tablet per os 4 times a day
2. 2 capsules by mouth every 6 hrs.
3. 2 of 500 mg. capsules orally every 4 hrs. preferable to 4 of 250 mg. capsules
4. 1/2 of 25 mg. tablet (in order to give least number of tablets possible) by mouth 4 times a day

143

5. 2 of 10 mg. and 1 of 5 mg. tablets orally 4 times a day or 5 of the 5 mg. tablets or 2 1/2 of 10 mg. tablets
6. 2 of 50 mg. capsules by mouth at hour of sleep as needed and may repeat 1 time (15 gr. = 1000 mg.)
7. 1/2 tablet orally 4 times a day (16 gr. = 1 Gr.)
8. 3 tablets orally 4 times a day
9. 2 tablets by mouth every 4 hrs. for 72 hrs. prior to surgery
10. 1 of 64 mg. and 1 of 32 mg. tablets by mouth 4 times a day (1 gr. = 64 mg.)
11. 1 of 1/120 gr. tablet by mouth 4 times a day (1 gr. = 60 mg.) or 1/132 (15 gr. = 1000 mg.)
12. 1 of 100 mg. tablet orally 3 times a day 15 gr. = 1000 mg.)

page 26–28
1. 5 ml. immediately by mouth
2. 10 ml. every 6 hrs. by mouth
3. 22.5 ml. orally every day
4. 5 ml. orally 3 times a day
5. 1 ml. of the 50 mg./ml. pediatric drops, 2 ml. of the 125 mg./5 ml. oral suspension, or 1 ml. of the 250 mg./5 ml. oral suspension orally four times a day
6. 2 drams or 8 ml. of the mixture (1 dram of each drug) orally 3 times a day
7. 2 cc. by mouth every 4 hrs. as needed
8. 0.4 ml. orally every day
9. 4 ml. orally every 4 hrs.
10. 4 ml. by mouth every 4 hrs. as needed (1 gr. = 64 mg.)
11. 10 ml. orally every 6 hrs.
12. 15 ml. by mouth 3 times a day

page 30–31
1. Dissolve 12.5 ml. (12.5 Gm.) or 3 tsp. of dextrose powder in 250 ml. of water and give orally 3 times a day.
2. Give 2/5 of a 30 mg. tablet, for example, by dissolving it in 30 ml. of water and giving 12 ml., by dissolving it in 20 ml. of water and giving 8 ml., or by dissolving it in 15 ml. of water and giving 6 ml. orally every 12 hours (or use 1/5th of the 60 mg. tablet or 6/50th of the 100 mg. tablet).
3. Add 2 ml. of water to a vial containing 60 mg. and give 0.5 ml. of the dissolved solution orally every 8 hours.
4. Give 5/16 of a 4 mg. tablet, for example, by dissolving it in 16 ml. of water and giving 5 ml. or by dissolving it in 32 ml. of water and giving 10 ml. orally 4 times a day.

page 34–36
1. Dissolve 9 ml. or 2 tsp. (9 Gm.) sodium chloride in 1 qt of tap water at correct temperature.
2. Dissolve 60 ml. or 2 oz. (60 Gm.) sodium bicarbonate in 2 qts. of sterile water (if available) at correct temperature.

3. Dissolve 2 of the 0.5 Gm. mercury bichloride tablets in 1000 ml. sterile distilled water.
4. Dissolve 1 of the 30 mg. gentian violet tablets in 1 oz. of water, preferably sterile. Using 2 of the 15 mg. or 3 of the 10 mg. tablets also is correct.
5. The 0.4 Gm. of drug needed is more than 1 of the 300 mg. (5 gr.) tablets. Therefore, dissolve 2 of the 5 gr. tablets in 6,000 ml. water (if calculating by using 2 tablets × 300 mg. each).
6. The amount of drug needed to make 1000 ml. solution is less than the 5 gr. which 1 tablet contains. Therefore, dissolve 1 of the 5 gr. tablets in 2400 ml. water (if calculating by using 1 tablet × 300 mg. each).
7. Dissolve 50 ml. (Gm.) boric acid crystals in 1000 ml. warm sterile water. (5% boric acid solution is saturated.)
8. Dissolve 2 ml. (2 Gm.) sodium perborate in 100 ml. water to use as mouth wash four times a day.

page 38-40
1. Use approximately 714 2/7 ml. of 70% alcohol and 1,285 5/7 ml. of tap water.
2. Use 60 ml. of the 5% dextrose and 60 ml. of water or 30 ml. of the 10% dextrose and 90 ml. of water.
3. Use 1 pt. of 70% isopropyl alcohol and 2 pts. of water.
4. Use 160 ml. 50% Lysol solution and 3840 ml. of water.
5. Use 1 part 1:100 Adrenalin and 9 parts water.
6. Use 10 ml. hydrogen peroxide (3%) and 20 ml. of water.
7. Use 200 ml. of 5% Dakin's solution and 1800 ml. of water.
8. Use 200 ml. of 5% boric acid solution and 300 ml. sterile water.

CHAPTER 3
PRACTICE PROBLEMS

1. 0.25 ml. subcutaneously every 8 hrs.
2. 3 ml. from 4 ml. (0.8 mg.) ampule (would be less expensive than 3 ml. from 2 of the 2 ml. [0.4 mg.] ampules) intramuscularly every day
3. 2 m. (1/8 ml. or 0.125 ml.) from 2 ml. (0.4 mg.) ampule intramuscularly immediately
4. 2 ml. (2 ampules) of the 10 mg./ml. solution intramuscularly immediately
5. 8 1/4 lbs. equals 3.75 kg. Dilute 1 ml. of epinephrine 1:1000 in 4 ml. sterile diluent and administer 0.1875 ml. subcutaneously immediately
6. 0.1 ml. intradermally at 9 a.m. tomorrow
7. 2 ml. intramuscularly immediately
8. 1.67 (1 2/3) cc. intramuscularly twice a day
9. 1 ml. hypodermically every 3 hrs. as needed for asthma
10. 2 ml. intramuscularly now; then 1 ml. every 6 hrs. as needed for nausea
11. 2 cc. intramuscularly 4 times a day as needed for asthma
12. 2 m. (0.125 ml.) hypodermically at 10 a.m. before surgery

1. Add 2 ml. diluent to the 1 Gm. vial and give 1.44 ml. I.M. every 4 hours. (500 mg.:1.2 ml. = 600 mg.:x ml.; 500 x = 720; x = 1.44 ml.) These directions indicate consistency of displacement.

2. *Note*: If the amount of drug is exactly the same as the label claim, the directions for reconstitution are in error, and the amounts of displacement, from top to bottom of the directions would be: − 0.2 ml., 0.0 ml., 0.2 ml., 0.5 ml. (not 2 times the displacement for 1/2 as much drug), and 1.2 ml. (not 4 times the displacement of 500 mg. and not 2 times the displacement for 1 Gm.).

or

LABEL CLAIM	AMOUNT DILUENT	WITH-DRAWABLE VOLUME	MG./ML. CONCEN-TRATION	DISPLACE-MENT	DISPLACE-MENT PER 125 MG.
125 mg.	1.2 ml.	1 ml.	125	− 0.2 ml.	− 0.2 ml.
250 mg.	1.0 ml.	1 ml.	250	0.0 ml.	0.0 ml.
500 mg.	1.8 ml.	2 ml.	250	0.2 ml.	0.05 ml.
1 Gm.	3.5 ml.	4 ml.	250	0.5 ml.	0.0625 ml.
2 Gm.	6.8 ml.	8 ml.	250	1.2 ml.	0.075 ml.

One can follow directions and add 1 ml. diluent to a 250 mg. vial and give 0.8 ml. (12.8 m.). Or, add 1 or 1.5 ml. of diluent (nurse selects amount) to a 250 mg. vial, measure the resulting total amount of solution and give four-fifths of the total amount.

$$\left(\frac{200 \text{ mg. ordered}}{250 \text{ mg. in vial}} = \frac{4}{5} \right).$$

3. The drug displacement when adding 2 ml. or 3 ml. to the 1 Gm. vial is consistent, 0.5 ml. However, if adding 3.6 ml. yields 4 ml., the displacement is 0.4 ml. Add 2 ml. diluent to the 1 Gm. vial and give the entire amount I.M. every six hours.

4. Add 4 ml. diluent to 2 Gm. vial and give three-fourths of the total amount which would be approximately 3.75 ml. (2 Gm.:5 ml. = 1.5 Gm.:x ml.; 2x = 7.5; x = 3.75 ml.)

5. Unless the amount of drug in each vial is different from the label claim, there is no way of knowing which of these directions, if any, may be correct. Add 5.7 ml. diluent to a 1 Gm. vial, measure the entire amount of the reconstituted solution and give three-fourths of the measured amount, or approximately 4.5 ml., probably in two sites. (250 mg.:1.5 ml. = 750 mg.:x ml.; 250x = 750 × 1.5; 250x = 1125; x = 4.5 ml.) To use one of the 250 mg. vials and one of the 500 mg. vials would cost the patient more than when using the 1 Gm. vial.

6. Add 2 ml. diluent and give 1.33 ml. I.M. stat and every 12 hours. (75 mg.:1 ml. = 100 mg.:x ml.; 75x = 100; x = 1.33 ml.)

7. Drug displacement for the 500 mg. vial is 0.2 ml.; for the 1 Gm. vial it is 0.4 ml. or 0.2 ml. per 500 mg. These are consistent. However, displace-

ment for the 2 Gm. vial is 1.0 ml. or 0.25 ml. per 500 mg. This must be questioned. Add 3 ml. of diluent to the 1 Gm. vial and give the entire amount, approximately 3.4 ml. I.M. every 8 hours.

8. Add 3 ml. diluent to 1 Gm. vial, measure the entire amount, return the total volume to the vial and give one-fourth of the total volume.

$$\left(\frac{250 \text{ mg.}}{1000 \text{ mg.}} = \frac{1}{4}\right)$$

9. Add 3 ml. diluent to the 1 Gm. vial, measure the entire amount and give three-fourths of the entire amount.

$$\left(\frac{750 \text{ mg.}}{1000 \text{ mg.}} = \frac{3}{4}\right)$$

10. Either one or both of the 125 mg. and 250 mg. vials do not have exactly 125 mg. and 250 mg. of drug in them, or there is an error in consistency of displacement by the drug, or 125 mg. of drug goes into solution without measurable displacement. As shown with this problem, there are inconsistencies of displacement for the 500 mg. and 1 Gm. vials when compared with the 2 Gm. vial. Add 1 ml. of diluent to 125 mg. vial, measure the entire amount, and give four-fifths of this amount.

$$\left(\frac{100 \text{ mg.}}{125 \text{ mg.}} = \frac{4}{5}\right)$$

11. Again we find apparent inconsistency of drug displacement:
    Adding 4 ml. diluent to 2 Gm. = 1 Gm./2.5 ml. or 5 ml. total, giving a displacement of 0.5 ml./Gm.
    Adding 6 ml. diluent to 3 Gm. = 1 Gm./2.5 ml. or 7.5 ml. total, giving a displacement of 0.5 ml./Gm.
    Adding 7.8 ml. diluent to 4 Gm. = 1 Gm./2.5 ml. or 10 ml. total, giving a displacement of 0.55 ml./Gm.
    This apparent error is probably within the margin of safety and the directions for reconstitution probably would be safe to use. Add 4 ml. diluent to 2 Gm. vial and give one-half, approximately 2.5 ml.

12. Again there is inconsistency in displacement:
    Adding 2 ml. diluent to 250 mg. = 125 mg./ml. or 2.0 ml. total, giving a displacement of 0.0 ml./250 mg.
    Adding 2 ml. diluent to 500 mg. = 225 mg./ml. or 2.2 ml. total, giving a displacement of 0.2 ml./500 mg. or 0.1 ml./250 mg.
    Adding 2.0 ml. diluent to 1 Gm. vial = 330 mg./ml. or 3.03 ml. total, giving a displacement of 1.03 ml./1 Gm. or 0.2575 ml./250 mg.
    Add 2 ml. to the 1 Gm. vial and give the entire amount I.M. every 6 hrs. and hope that this is within the 10% margin of error.

page 65-67
1. Using a tuberculin syringe, measure 0.2 ml. (1.6 m.) of 100 U. regular insulin and give 20 minutes before meals three times a day.

2. Using a tuberculin syringe measure 1.8 ml. (2.88 m.) of 100 U. P.Z.I. insulin. Since 50 U and 100 U. insulin syringes are available, one of them should be used. Draw up 100 U. P.Z.I. insulin to the 18 U. mark on either syringe and administer at 4 p.m. each day.
3. Using a tuberculin syringe measure 0.05 ml. (0.8 m.) 100 U. regular insulin and administer 20 minutes before meals three times a day.
4. Use a 50 U. or 100 U. insulin syringe and draw up 24 U. regular insulin on either syringe and administer 20 minutes before meals three times a day.
5. Use a 100 U. insulin syringe, put 45 U. of air into the N.P.H. insulin vial, withdraw the needle; put 24 U. of air into the regular insulin vial, draw out 24 U. of the 100 U. regular insulin; then draw insulin out of the 100 U. N.P.H. insulin vial to the 69 U. mark (24 U. regular plus 45 U. N.P.H. equals 69 U. total measurement). Administer 1 hour before breakfast tomorrow.
6. Use a 50 U. or 100 U. insulin syringe and draw up 100 U. Lente insulin to the 46 U. mark. If a tuberculin syringe is used, draw insulin to the 0.46 ml. (7.36 m.) mark and administer 1 hour before breakfast each day.
7. Use a tuberculin syringe and draw 100 U. Ultralente insulin to the 0.65 ml. (10.4 m.) mark and administer 1 hour before breakfast tomorrow.
8. Use a tuberculin syringe and draw 100 U. Semilente insulin to the 0.18 ml. (2.88 m.) mark and administer one-half hour before breakfast every day.
9. Use either the 0.5 ml. or 1 ml. 100 U. insulin syringe and draw 100 U. Ultralente to the 46 U. mark and administer 1 hour before breakfast each day.

page 84–91
1. 62.5 or 62 or 63 drops per minute
2. 111 1/9 or 111 drops per minute
3. 41 2/3 or 42 drops per minute (no more than 20–25 Eq KCl/hr)
4. 31 1/4 or 31 drops per minute
5. 30.68 or 31 drops per minute
6. 16 2/3 or 17 drops per minute
7. 27 7/9 or 28 drops per minute
8. 26 2/3 or 27 drops per minute
9. Withdraw 20 ml. of fluid from a 500 ml. bag of D = 5 = W and add 20 ml. aminophyllin (250 mg.:10 ml. = 500 mg.:x ml.; x = 20 ml.). Regulate the IVAC to flow at 30 ml./hr. (500 mg.:500 ml. = 30 mg.:x ml.; 500 x = 15,000; x = 30 ml.; or, 1 mg.:1 ml. = 30 mg.:x ml.; x = 30 ml.).
10. Since 100 ml. should run 12.5 hours, the nurse decides to put the aminophylline in 100 ml. D-5-W (1 mg.:1 ml. = 8 mg. (per hr.):x ml.; x = 8 ml./hr., then, 8 ml.:1 hr. = 100 ml.:x hr.; 8 x = 100; x = 12.5 hrs.). Add 4 ml. of the aminophylline 250 mg./10 ml. to the 100 ml. D-5-W (1 mg.:1 ml. = x mg.:100 ml.; x = 100 mg., then, 250 mg.:10 ml. = 100 mg.: x ml.; 250 x = 1,000; x = 4 ml.).
11. Put 49.75 ml. of N.S. and 0.25 ml. (25 U.) of Regular Insulin 100 U/ml. in Harvard infusor 50 ml. syringe. Set infusor at 2 ml./hr. (25 U.:50 ml. =

1.0 U.:x ml.; 25 x = 50; x = 2 ml.). There will be 1 U. of insulin in 2 ml. of fluid at end of 24 hrs.

12. According to hospital policy or practice, for the length of time an I.V. bottle or bag should hang, one of the three sizes of containers will be infusing. Use 1 ml. of Valium (5 mg./ml.). It will be easier to give this drug in a minimum of 1 minute if approximately 5–10 ml. of diluent is added to the valium before it is injected slowly into the flashball near the venipuncture needle.

13. Add 0.5 ml. of Neo-Synephrine (10 mg.:1 ml. = 5 mg.:x ml.; 10 x = 5; x = 0.5 ml.) into 500 ml. of D-5-W and mix. Regulate the IMED at 3 ml./hr. (5,000 mcg. (5 mg.):500 ml. = 0.5 mcg. x ml. (per min.); 5,000 x = 250; x = 0.05 ml./min., then, 0.05 ml.:1 min. = x ml.:60 min.; x = 3 ml./hr.)

14. At the end of the hour when the drug is to be given add 1.5 ml. genta-mycin (20 mg.:2 ml. = 15 mg.:x ml.; 20 x = 30; x = 1.5 ml.) to the Solu-set. Add I.V. solution to a total of 15 ml. (not 15 ml. plus 10 ml.) in the Soluset. Continue flow at 15 ml./hr. or 15 gtts./min. for 1 hour. When Soluset empties add 25 ml. (15 ml. plus 10 ml. reserve) to Soluset and continue flow at 15 gtts./min.

15. Putting a 24-hour supply of drug in a Harvard syringe pump is a com-mon practice in some hospitals. For the 50 ml. to run 24 hours, the rate would need to be approximately 2 ml./hr. At 2 ml./hr. the infusion would run 25 hrs. Heparin 12,500 U. are needed (500 U.:2 ml. = x U.: 50 ml.; 2 x = 25,000; x = 12,500 U.; or, 500 U.:1 hr. = x U.:25 hrs.; x = 12,500 U.). To get heparin 12,500 use 0.83 ml. of the 15,000 U./ml. hepa-rin (15,000 U.:1 ml. = 12,500 U.:x ml.; 15,000 x = 12,500; x = 0.83 ml. of the 15,000 U./ml. heparin and fill with I.V. solution to 50 ml. Set the Harvard infusor at 2 ml./hr., leaving 2 ml. at the end of 24 hrs.

16. Use 0.3 ml. of Vira-A (200 mg.:1 ml. = 60 mg.:x ml.; 200 x = 60; x = 0.3 ml.). Put 0.3 ml. of this drug in a minimum of 133 ml. of I.V. solution (2.22 ml.:1 mg. = x ml.:60 mg.; x = 133.2 ml.). If 0.3 ml. of drug were put into the Buretrol and it was filled to 150 ml. mark, the IMED would need to be set at 6.25 ml./hr. (150 ml.:24 hrs. = x ml.:1 hr.; 24 x = 150; x = 6.25 ml.). The machine can only be set at 6.2 or 6.3 ml./hr., so fill the Buretrol to 148.8 ml. and set the IMED at 6.2 ml./hr. (6.2 ml.:1 hr. = x ml.:24 hrs.; x = 144 ml.). Warm solution according to hospital practice.

17. Put 250 mg. of the drug into a Harvard syringe and fill it to 50 ml. Regu-late infusor at 3 ml./hr. (1000 mcg.:1 mg. = 250 mcg.:x mg.; 1000 x = 250; x = 0.25 mg./min. or 15 mg./hr., then, 250 mg.:50 ml. = 15 mg.:x ml.; 250 x = 750; x = 3 ml./hr., or, 250 mcg.:1 min. = x mcg.:60 min.; x = 15,000 mcg./hr. = 15 mg./hr., then 250 mg.:50 ml. = 15 mg.:x ml.; 250 x = 750; x = 3 ml./hr.).

18. Put drug in minimum of 12.5 ml. of fluid. Add contents of 500 mg. vial of drug to a 50 ml. P.B. bag of I.V. solution, connect secondary set to P.B. bag and into secondary portal on primary tubing. Elevate P.B. bag above primary I.V. solution and continue flow at 40 ml./hr. or 10 gtts./min. (15 gtts.:1 ml. = x gtts.:40 ml.; x = 600 gtts/hr., then, 600

gtts.:60 min. = x gtts.:1 min.; $60 x = 600$; $x = 10$ gtts./min., or 15 gtts. × 40 ml./hr. = 600 gtts./hr., then 600 gtts. ÷ 60 min. = 10 gtts./min.).

19. Reconstitute drug as directed and withdraw 5 ml. of drug (1000 mg.: 10 ml. = 500 mg.:x ml.; $1000 x = 5000$; $x = 5$ ml.). Label and refrigerate the unused portion of the drug. To make it easier to give the drug in a minimum of 1 minute, additional diluent, e.g., 5 ml., could be added for a total of 10 ml. Carry out usual heparin lock flush procedure and give the drug in 1 minute or more.

20. Put 20 ml. (5 Gm.) of drug and 30 ml. I.V. solution in 50 ml. syringe. Regulate flow at 10 ml./hr. (5 Gm.:50 ml. = 1 Gm.:x ml.; $5 x = 50$; $x = 10$ ml./hr.).

21. Reconstitute 1 Gm. vial of drug with 2 ml. diluent and withdrawn 2.4 ml. (500 mg.:1.2 ml. = 1000 mg.:x ml.; $500 x = 1200$; $x = 2.4$ ml.). Add the drug to a 50 ml. P.B. bag of solution. Regulate the I.V. flow at 25 gtts./min. (50 ml. × 10 gtts./ml. = 500 gtts. ÷ 20 min. = 25 gtts./min.).

22. Use 2 ml. ampule of drug and withdraw 1.33 ml. (150 mg.:1 ml. = 200 mg.:x ml.; $150 x = 200$; $x = 1.33$ ml.). Put the drug into a 50 ml. P.B. bag of the appropriate I.V. solution, connect secondary I.V. tubing, elevate the P.B. bag, and run the medication fluid into the last portal on the primary tubing at 50 ml./hr. or 50 gtts./min.

23. This drug will be most stable with 1 Gm. in a minimum of 20 ml. (50 mg.:1 ml. = 1000 mg.:x ml.; $50 x = 1000$, $x = 20$ ml.) or in a maximum of 100 ml. (10 mg.:1 ml. = 1000 mg.: x ml.; $10 x = 1000$; $x = 100$ ml.). Therefore, put contents of 1 Gm. vial of reconstituted drug into 50 ml. P.B. bag of solution, connect Abbot I.V. set to bag and heparin lock after flushing lock. Regulate flow at 12 or 13 gtts./min. (50 ml. × 15 gtts./ml. = 750 gtts./hr.; 750 gtts. ÷ 60 min. = 12.5 gtts./min.).

24. Withdraw 3.125 ml. of drug (16 mg.:1 ml. = 50 mg.:x ml.; $16 x = 50$; $x = 3.125$ ml.). Add this drug to the Soluset by syringe and needle and add D-5-W to at least the 78 ml. mark (80 mg.:125 ml. = 50 mg.:x ml.; $80 x = 6250$; x 78.125 ml.) and regulate flow at 78 gtts./min. If Soluset was filled to 100 ml. the flow should be 100 gtts./min. (with microdrip chambers, the ml./hr. = gtts./min.).

CHAPTER 4
PRACTICE PROBLEMS

1. BSA = 0.88 m² via nomogram; $\dfrac{0.88 \times 1.0}{1.7} = \dfrac{0.88}{1.7} = 0.518$ Gm. = safe dose for this child; give 1 tablet by mouth q. 4 hours.

2. BSA = 0.4 m² via normal height for weight chart; $\dfrac{0.4 \text{ m}^2 \times 5 \text{ gr.}}{1.7} = \dfrac{2}{1.7} = 1.18$, and, $\dfrac{0.4 \text{ m}^2 \times 10 \text{ gr.}}{1.7} = \dfrac{4}{1.7} = 2.35$, so, 1.18 gr. to 2.35 gr. is safe dose range for this baby; give gr. 1 tablet every 4 hrs. Even though use of BSA for infants less than 10 kilograms may yield exces-

sive dosages, this is the only method that can be used with the information available.

3. 22 lbs. = 10 kg.; 50 mg.:1 kg. = x mg.:10 kg.; x = 500 mg. The safe range equals the amount ordered, so reconstitute a 1 Gm. vial of Mezlin, withdraw one-half of the solution, further dilute as directed, and give I.V. every 4 hours.

4. BSA = 0.76 m² via nomogram; $\dfrac{0.76 \times 24}{1.7} = \dfrac{18.24}{1.7} = 10.73$ Gm. = safe daily dose; 2 Gm. every 6 hours = 8 Gm./day. Reconstitute a 2 Gm. vial as directed and give I.V. every 6 hrs.

5. BSA via nomogram = 1.04 m²; $\dfrac{1.04 \times 100}{1.7} = \dfrac{104}{1.7} = 61.18$ mg./day = maximum safe dosage for this child; give one-half of a 25 mg. tablet four times a day for a total of 50 mg./day.

6. Weight = 29.1 kg.; 0.7 mg.:1 kg. = x mg.:29.1 kg.; x = 20.37 mg./day compared with the 50 mg./day ordered. This is another example where different directions yield different safe dosages. Assess all factors before giving this child the ordered dosage or checking with the physician.

7. Using the first directions, 40 mg.:1 kg. = x mg.:8 kg.; x = 320 mg./day maximum dose compared with the 300 mg. ordered, therefore the order is reasonable. However, using the second directions, the BSA = 0.41 m² via nomogram; 450 mg.:1 m² = x mg.:0.41 m²; x = 184.5 mg./day maximum dose which is less than the 300 mg./day ordered. The third directions for a minimum of 300 mg./day make this order safe to give 0.5 ml., further diluted as directed, I.V. every 6 hrs.

8. 20 kg. = 44 lbs.; BSA via normal height for weight chart is 0.8 m². Using the adult doses, $\dfrac{0.8 \text{ m}^2 \times 1.0 \text{ mg.}}{1.7} = \dfrac{0.8}{1.7} = 0.47$ mg., which would be the average daily digitalizing dose for this child; and $\dfrac{0.8 \times 0.5}{1.7} =$ $\dfrac{0.4}{1.7} = 0.235$ mg. would be the average daily maintenance dose for this child, or respectively, 0.235 mg. and 0.1175 mg. twice a day. The ordered dose is considerably less than these amounts. Therefore, 0.5 ml. of the 0.1 mg./ml. available drug should be further diluted and given I.V. twice a day.

9. If 1 kg.:2.2 lbs. = x kg.:40 lbs; 2.2 x = 40; x 18.18 kg. = this child's weight. Thus 1000 mg.:1 kg. = x mg.:18.18 kg.; x = 1818 mg./day or 454.5 mg. every 6 hrs., less than the amount ordered, but the amount ordered is less than the amount recommended with mild renal failure. Reconstitute one of the 500 mg. vials, further dilute, and give I.V. every 6 hrs.

10. *Note*: The amount of drug/kg./day to be given varies with the disease condition. See directions in Problem 9; 100 mg.:1 kg. = x mg.:8.8 kg.; x = 880 mg./day or 220 mg. every 6 hrs.; and 150 mg.:1 kg. = x mg.: 8.8 kg.; x = 1320 mg./day or 330 mg. every 6 hrs.; the ordered dose is

reasonable. Reconstitute as directed and calculate the amount of drug to be further diluted and given I.V. every 6 hrs.

11. Ampicillin: 200 mg.:1 kg. = x mg.:4.4 kg.; x = 880 mg./day = 146.67 mg. every 4 hrs., more than the ordered dose, so, reconstitute a 125 mg. vial and give entire amount I.V. every 4 hrs.
Chloramphenicol: 100 mg.:1 kg. = x mg.:4.4 kg.; x = 440 mg./day = 110 mg. q.6h. more than the ordered dose, so, reconstitute as directed and give 1 ml. I.V. every 6 hrs.

12. 2.2 lbs.:1 kg. = 75 lbs.:x kg.; x = 34.09 kg.; 80 mg.:1 kg. = x mg.:34 kg.; x = 2720 mg./day = maximum of 680 mg. every 6 hrs. Reconstitute 500 mg. Cefadyl with 1 ml. diluent and give 1.2 ml., further diluted, I.V. every 6 hrs.

CHAPTER 5
REVIEW PROBLEMS

1. 10 gr. (60 mg. = 1 gr.)
2. 0.05 Gm.
3. 100 mg. (15 gr. = 1000 mg.)
4. 1 1/2 gr. (15 gr. = 1000 mg.)
5. Administer 2.25 ml. (if using 1 gr. = 60 mg.) intramuscularly immediately or 2.4375 mi. (if using 1 gr. = 65 mg.).
6. 20 5/6 or 21 drops per minute
7. Draw lente insulin to the 50 U mark of the 100 U syringe.
8. Administer 2 of the 5 gr. ASA tablets orally every 3 to 4 hrs. as needed. (15 or 16 gr. = 1 Gm.)
9. Administer 0.8 (12.8 m.) ml. epinephrine 1:2000 hypodermically every 3 hrs. as needed.
10. Use 357 1/7 ml. of 70% alcohol and 642 6/7 ml. of water.
11. Administer 2 ml. Nembutal, 1.5 ml. Demerol, and 1 ml. atropine hypodermically on call.
12. Administer 0.6 ml. Kantrex intramuscularly every 12 hrs.
13. Give 12 ml. (if using 32 ml. per oz.) Kaon 3 times a day.
14. Add 18 Gm. (1 tbsp. or 4 tsp.) of salt to 2 qts. of tap water at the proper temperature and administer.
15. Add 3.6 ml. sterile diluent to vial, dissolve drug, label vial "250,000 U./ ml.," and give 1.6 ml. intramuscularly every 4 hrs.
16. Give two ii$\overline{ss}$ gr. tablets (60 mg. = 1 gr.)
17. To give 1/2 gr. give 1/2 dram or 2 ml. (60 mg. = 1 gr.)
18. Give 3/4 ml. or 0.75 ml. or 12 m.
19. Use a tuberculin syringe and give 0.15 ml. (2.4 m.) regular insulin and 0.3 ml. (4.8 m.) of N.P.H. insulin.
20. Administer 1 of the 30 mg. phenobarbital sodium tablets orally 4 times a day.
21. Prepare drug solution; withdraw 0.05 ml. in tuberculin syringe; add diluent to a total of 1 ml. and put on Auto-Syringe; and set it to deliver 1 ml. in 30 minutes.

22. Dissolve 1 phenobarbital sodium tablet in 30 ml. water and give 5 ml. by mouth immediately.

23. Using a 6 ml. syringe, add 1 ml. diluent to 125 mg. vial; withdraw 0.8 ml. of reconstituted drug solution; add diluent to get 5 ml. drug solution; and give into proper portal at rate of 1 ml./minute.

24. 2.2 lbs.:1 kg. = 24 lbs.:x kg.; 2.2 x = 24; x = 10.91 kg.; 20 mg.:1 kg. = x mg.:10.9 kg.; x = 218 mg./day = 72.67 mg. every 8 hrs., just slightly less than the ordered amount. Using nomogram BSA = 0.5 m^2;

$$\frac{0.5 \; m^2 \times 250 \; mg.}{1.7} = x; x = \frac{125}{1.7}; x = 73.53 \; mg.,$$ slightly less than the ordered dose.

25. 0.5 mg.:1 lb. = x mg.:45 lbs., x = 22.5 mg., more than the ordered dose so give 0.8 ml. I.M. stat.

26. Reconstitute ampicillin as directed, add to 50 ml. D-5-W, and infuse piggyback at a rate of at least 8 1/3 or 9 gtts./min. in order to give the drug within an hour. Add 2.67 ml. clindamycin to 100 ml. D-5-W (to keep the concentration less than 300 mg./50 ml.) and give piggyback at 16 2/3 or 17 gtts./minute in order to give in 1 hour. (These drugs are incompatible so one should not be given immediately after the other.)

27. Inject 0.5 ml. of the 100 U heparin into the flashball while temporarily occluding the I.V. tubing above the injection site.

28. Regulate the rate of flow at 33 1/3 or 33 drops/minute unless a slower rate is indicated.

29. Use a tuberculin syringe. A total measurement of 0.45 ml. (0.35 ml. lente insulin and 0.1 ml. regular insulin) is needed. Draw 0.1 ml. of regular insulin into the syringe then draw N.P.H. insulin to the 0.45 ml. mark. In minims, the total measurement would be 7.2 minims, 5.6 m. of lente insulin and 1.6 m. of regular insulin.

30. Since there are no directions for reconstituting the Prostaphlin, add enough diluent to dissolve the drug, measure the entire amount, replace one-half into the vial, label the vial correctly, and add the other one-half to 62.5 ml. I.V. solution in the drip chamber. (To provide a concentration of 0.5 to 2.0 mg./ml., a maximum of 250 ml. of diluent to a minimum of 62.5 ml. of diluent is needed. The drug is to be given at no more than 50 mg./hour or in a minimum of 2 1/2 hours. At its present rate of 24 ml./hour, 62.5 ml. would run 2.6 hours.) Continue flow at 24 gtts./minute.

31. 0.6 Gm. = 10 gr. (60 mg. = 1 gr.) therefore give two of the v gr. aspirin tablets.

32. Give 2 ml. of the 1/8 gr./ml. morphine.

33. 10 Gms. of boric acid are needed to make 500 ml. of 2% solution; 200 ml. of the 5% boric acid solution contains 10 Gm. of boric acid. Add 200 ml. of 5% boric acid solution to 300 ml. of water to get 500 ml. of 2% boric acid solution.

34. 400 Gms. of sodium bicarbonate powder are needed to make 2 liters of 20% boric acid solution.

INDEX

An *italic* number indicates a figure. A "t" indicates a table.

25mg / 5000 cc

5000mg / 0

6mg / 0 / X

25mg / +

4000 mg/cc / 0

25mg

4mg / 0 / X

25mg / 250 cc / 0

25mg / 25

100mg/cc / 0 / 25

50cc / 0

4mg

40cc / 0

250 / 1000